Clinical Management Of
Temporomandibular Disorders

Also by Welden E. Bell:
OROFACIAL PAINS: DIFFERENTIAL DIAGNOSIS

CLINICAL MANAGEMENT OF TEMPOROMANDIBULAR DISORDERS

Welden E. Bell, D.D.S.
Clinical Professor of Oral Surgery
The University of Texas
Southwestern Medical School at Dallas
Dallas, Texas

YEAR BOOK MEDICAL PUBLISHERS, INC.
CHICAGO · LONDON

Reprinted, January 1983
Reprinted, July 1983

Library of Congress Cataloging in Publication Data

Bell, Welden E.
     Clinical management of temporomandibular disorders.

     Includes bibliographical references and index.
     1.   Temporomandibular joint—Diseases.
2.   Temporomandibular joint.   I.   Title.   [DNLM:
1.   Joint diseases.   2.   Mandibular condyle.
3.   Temporomandibular joint. WU 140 B435c]
RK470.B44   617'.522   81-16487
ISBN 0-8151-0652-1   AACR2

To honor the memory of
HARRY SICHER
who very patiently taught me
the biomechanics of the
craniomandibular articulation

CONTENTS

PREFACE

A CONFUSING IDEA about temporomandibular function permeates the dental literature—the idea that the mandibular condyle, with an interposed meniscus, articulates with the temporal bone. This, of course, is the way it looks when viewed radiographically. For many years, however, it has been evident that this joint is not that simple.

Since 1949,[1] the temporomandibular joint has been described as a true compound joint composed of a lower hinge portion that slides against the articular eminence above. Since 1951,[2] collateral ligaments attaching the articular disc to the condyle have been recognized. Since 1964,[3] it has been known that the articulating parts of this joint, like all other synovial joints, must remain in sharp contact at all times in order to function normally. Why, then, should this joint be so poorly understood?

The purpose of this book is to dispel the mystery that has bred confusion, and some controversy, in the management of masticatory complaints. The objective is to portray as clearly as possible the principles of biomechanics that govern this joint, to refine them in the light of experimental documentation, and to bring them into a clinical setting that can serve as a better foundation for the diagnosis and treatment of complaints in this important area.

One key to understanding masticatory function is that the articular disc is not a passive meniscus separating the articulating bones, as in the knee joint. Rather, it is an active, dynamic part of the joint, serving as a third bone in a true compound joint. Attached to the lateral poles of the mandibular condyle by collateral ligaments, the articular disc is powered to function independently of both condyle and temporal bone—an anatomically unique and functionally distinctive feature of the temporomandibular joint. This structure rotates anteriorly (by the superior head of the lateral pterygoid muscle) when the condyle moves posteriorly during power strokes and maximum intercuspation. It rotates posteriorly (by action of the elastic su-

---

[1]Sicher H.: *Oral Anatomy*. St. Louis, C.V. Mosby Co., 1949.

[2]Sicher H.: Functional anatomy of the temporomandibular joint, in Sarnat B.G. (ed.): *The Temporomandibular Joint*. Springfield, Ill., Charles C Thomas, Publisher, 1951, pp. 3–40.

[3]Sicher H.: Functional anatomy of the temporomandibular joint, in Sarnat B.G. (ed.): *The Temporomandibular Joint*, ed. 2. Springfield, Ill., Charles C Thomas, Publisher, 1964, pp. 28–58.

perior retrodiscal lamina) when the condyle moves anteriorly into the forward phase of translatory cycles. The independent movements of this "third bone" are not incidental; they are necessary functions—necessary to maintain sharp contact between the articulating parts of this synovial joint and thus ensure normal joint function. This is significantly different from the conventional concept of articulation of bone against bone with an interposed meniscus. It brings the disc alive in its true functional role in masticatory movements. Surely a more lucid understanding of joint function and dysfunction will evolve as this concept of articular disc action becomes better understood, for in it lies many answers to the peculiar symptoms and antics that this joint displays, to the bewilderment of dentists everywhere.

The method of diagnosis and treatment embodied in this book rests on fundamental biomechanics originally conceived in large part by Harry Sicher. Although some earlier concepts have undergone modification, others have been reinforced by experimental evidence, especially in the field of muscle physiology. This concept of management has evolved during 40 years of clinical practice. Time has refined it to its present form.

It is my earnest wish that these principles and guidelines may help others find a way toward more effective clinical management of temporomandibular disorders.

WELDEN E. BELL

1 / A Problem for Clinical Dentistry

THROUGHOUT HISTORY, and even today, temporomandibular complaints have been troublesome for doctors to manage well. First medical doctors and subsequently dentists have tried to cope with such problems. On the whole, however, clinical results have been less than satisfying. Frequently the patient is disappointed and the doctor is frustrated. But the accumulation of scientific knowledge about the structures and mechanisms involved has been quite satisfactory. It appears, therefore, that the difficulty lies not so much in lack of basic knowledge as in failure to apply that information at a clinical level.

DEFINING THE PROBLEM

Disorders of the masticatory system are the very substance of dentistry. Clinical management of the dentition proper comprises the major day-to-day duties of the practicing dentist. Management of the masticatory system, however, does not end with the presence, normal structural form, proper alignment, and harmonious occlusion of teeth. The dentition proper represents only the working ends of the apparatus, the tools by which mastication is accomplished, not the system itself.

Prehension, incising, grinding, and swallowing foods are vital body functions. The same is true of respiration and speech, in which the oral structures participate importantly. The mechanisms of oral communication and orofacial expression make social intercourse pleasant and profitable. Chronologically, the oral cavity is the initial organ of sexual expression and throughout life never completely loses this emotional association. The mouth and orofacial structures constitute a region of unusual emotional significance that remains sensitive to threat and responsive to clinical management.

The masticatory system is a complex one indeed. During the many patterns of action required for the preparation of food prior to deglutition, the intricate mechanics involved in the articulation of tooth surfaces (occlusal function) is a study in itself. Mastication calls on an integrated and precisely coordinated biologic system of bones, joints, ligaments, muscles, vessels, nerves, and glands that extends from the lips to the larynx and from the teeth to the esophagus. This system can be affected by disorders and com-

1

plications without number. It is the purpose of this book to consider in depth one group of disorders of this complex system: the so-called temporomandibular disorders.

More precisely, the objectives of this book are:

1. To consider the anatomical and physiologic factors involved in normal functioning of the masticatory apparatus, other than occlusion per se.

2. To consider departures from normal structural and functional behavior of the masticatory apparatus, other than problems of occlusion per se.

3. The clinical identification of such departures from normal.

4. To establish guidelines for the clinical management of temporomandibular disorders that constitute such departures from normal.

Historical Background

The historical record of the clinical management of temporomandibular disorders is colorful indeed. Many patients with complaints of this type have found themselves in a medical no-man's-land, in that orthopedists have seemed unable to grasp the full significance of masticatory physiology or cope with its impact on disorders of this type, and dentists who undertake management do so without benefit of adequate training and experience in orthopedic medicine. In retrospect, it appears that this clinical dilemma is really a spinoff from the unfortunate separation of the two professions.

In 1934, the otolaryngologist Costen[1] drew attention to the syndrome that bears his name by concluding that lost vertical dimension in the chewing apparatus was chiefly responsible for the complaints. It was a case of astute observation from which an improper conclusion was drawn. Costen correctly observed that disengagement of the occlusion did benefit many of his patients, just as the restriction of traumatic activity in general is known to ameliorate other types of orthopedic complaints. From this observation, however, he improperly assumed that the disengaging material placed between the teeth yielded benefit *because it opened the bite*. He concluded that the chief cause of the complaint was a "closed bite." As a result, the treatment in vogue for many years was the empirical application of various forms of bite-raising dental procedures.

Although the expected results were disappointing, the belief that occlusion is the key to temporomandibular complaints dominated dental practitioners' thinking until the present. Thus, preoccupied as the dental profession has been with occlusion as the dominant etiologic factor and occlusal therapy as the chief form of treatment, the gap between the professions has widened until the problem has come to rest in the lap of dentistry. Unfortunately, most practicing dentists, untrained in orthopedics and unschooled in diagnostic techniques, have not been able to manage the problem effectively, nor has the dental educational system met the challenge thus presented.

Temporomandibular therapy since the time of Costen has been largely empirical and oftentimes controversial. Different modalities of treatment have dominated at different times. The profession has witnessed a host of temporarily popular procedures, such as bite-raising, injection of sclerosing solutions into the joints, rehabilitation and reconstruction of the dentition, use of occlusal pivots, surgical removal of the articular disc, occlusal equilibration, use of interocclusal appliances, orthodontics, surgical condylectomy, physiotherapy, injection of cortisone into the joints, muscle relaxant therapy, psychotherapy and tension control, surgical repair of displaced articular discs, and applied kinesiology. Most forms of therapy have concentrated on a particular component of the masticatory apparatus: the dentition, the joints, the musculature. The popularity of any particular treatment modality seemed to bear little relationship to the considerably more orderly accumulation of basic scientific knowledge of the masticatory system. *Important as the dentition is with regard to masticatory function and dysfunction, the passing of time has demonstrated that there is no substitute for a full understanding of the entire masticatory system.* The historical, controversial management of such disorders likely stems from consideration of single components of the masticatory apparatus without regard for the whole system as a functioning unit. History should teach that it is expedient to go back to basics and assimilate on a clinical level the mass of scientific knowledge that has been available for many years, and which should be the basis for the rational diagnosis and effective treatment of temporomandibular disorders.

Prior to Costen's work, anatomists described the structures of the joint in general terms, with little reference to masticatory function. With the publication of his *Oral Anatomy* in 1949,[11] Sicher emerged as the dominant figure. His book provided accurate descriptions of the components of the masticatory apparatus, correlating the anatomical structures with the requirements of function. In 1954, Rees, the British anatomist, added to Sicher's brilliant work.[10] Had Rees lived to note the later work of Krogh-Poulsen and Moelhave in 1957,[5] perhaps some of the confusion of recent years might not have taken place at all. Du Brul[3] has added significantly to Sicher's monumental work.

During this same period, giant strides were made in the understanding of the evolution, embryology, growth and development, functional remodeling, and histopathology of the masticatory apparatus. For this, the profession is indebted to many dedicated researchers from a variety of disciplines.

A better understanding of pain mechanisms and muscle physiology has contributed significantly to the knowledge of masticatory dysfunctions and disorders. The muscular genesis of pain, the secondary effects of deep pain, the modulation of pain impulses, and the discovery of an endogenous antinociceptive system have opened new avenues of thought on masticatory pains. Electromyographic studies have done much to elucidate muscle function, to isolate and identify the action of specific masticatory muscles with the different jaw movements, and to augment the comprehension of what takes place in the process of incising and grinding foods.

More uniform terminology, improved classification of orofacial pain syndromes, more accurate categorization of temporomandibular disorders, and enlightened examining techniques have streamlined the clinical task of identifying disorders of the temporomandibular joints and masticatory musculature. The accumulation of clinical data on etiologic factors, particularly those relevant to abusive habits, bruxism, emotional stress, trauma, and occlusal discrepancies, has given better insight into cause and prevention. Interdisciplinary cooperation in management is doing much to develop guidelines for a rational approach to the whole problem.

There is now a sizable mass of reliable, factual, scientific information available to researchers and clinicians alike. Using this information, unified concepts of normal masticatory function can be formed, criteria for the recognition of masticatory dysfunctions can be established, and effective measures to alleviate temporomandibular complaints can be developed. There is no longer any valid reason for divisive, conflicting, and mutually exclusive concepts of what constitutes normal masticatory function. Purely empirical and trial-and-error therapy are no longer justifiable. Precise differential diagnosis and rational, predictable treatment methods can bring management of most temporomandibular disorders within the grasp of knowledgeable practitioners of dentistry.

Responsibility for Management

Ordinarily, complaints involving the masticatory system are presented to the dentist directly by the patient or by the referring physician on the assumption that they relate to the dentition. Some complaints are not attended by pain or discomfort, the disorder being wholly that of dysfunction. Such complaints include (1) restriction of jaw movement that interferes with opening the mouth or making usual chewing movements, (2) abnormal noises or strange sensations during jaw movements, and (3) a sudden alteration in the bite. Some complaints consist of pain only—discomfort with chewing and jaw movements. Most complaints, however, have components of dysfunction and pain in myriad combinations. The management of all such complaints involves diagnosis and treatment.

DIAGNOSIS.—It is a serious mistake to assume that the presenting symptoms automatically indicate the proper category into which the particular complaint should fall. Nor do they signify the seriousness of the problem or responsiveness to treatment. It is the responsibility of the examining dentist to make a diagnosis prior to undertaking definitive treatment. An accurate diagnosis is the first step in the treatment of any disorder, and the process cannot be abridged.

The diagnosis of disorders of the masticatory system requires the services of a dentist knowledgeable in pain and oriented toward masticatory function. Only he has the training and expertise to trace pain sources and judge masticatory function. It is the professional obligation of every dentist who undertakes the management of such disorders to make himself proficient in these areas.

A diagnosis should (1) identify and classify the disorder properly, (2) establish the reason for dysfunction and the source of pain, (3) determine the etiology, if at all possible, and (4) provide a basis for prognosis in the light of effective therapy.

TREATMENT.—Although the dentist is responsible for the diagnosis, subsequent treatment may or may not rest in his hands. If etiologic factors in the case are exclusively related to conditions amenable to dental treatment, then the responsibility for therapy should remain the dentist's. Interdisciplinary dental cooperative effort, however, may be needed to ensure a successful outcome. Some temporomandibular disorders are associated with conditions that are not responsive to dental treatment measures. Management of these conditions should be done by an appropriate medical practitioner or by a cooperative interdisciplinary team.

Preliminary consultations prior to definitive therapy may do much to smooth the clinical course and ensure the outcome of complex masticatory conditions.

SYNOVIAL JOINTS

The word *articulation,* meaning the place of junction between two discrete objects, is used in orthopedic nomenclature to designate the place of union or junction between two or more bones of the skeleton. Such articulations are commonly called *joints.* Joints are classified as *synarthrodial* or *diarthrodial.*

In *synarthrodial or fibrous joints,* the parts are united by fibrous tissue. When the intervening fibrous tissue is continuous, the joint is referred to as a *suture.* Some common sutures are those of the cranial bones and the pubic symphysis. When the bones are connected by ligaments only, the joint is referred to as *syndesmosis;* an example is the tibiofibular articulation. When the fibrous joint is composed of a conical process inserted into a socket-like portion, it is referred to as *gomphosis*. The teeth in the alveolar process form such a joint.

Diarthrodial joints are discontinuous articulations that permit greater freedom of movement between the united parts. The articulating surfaces are composed of a tissue able to sustain compression and movement simultaneously, a condition that precludes the presence of blood vessels and nerve receptors in the pressure-bearing areas. Metabolic and nutritional requirements of such nonvascularized tissue are provided by surface contact of joint fluid, called *synovial fluid*. The presence of synovial fluid requires that the articular surfaces be encapsulated to confine it. The inner surface of the capsule is composed of a specialized connective tissue that secretes the synovial fluid, the *synovial membrane*. Because of this structural arrangement imposed on movable joints by the demands of simultaneous compression and movement, diarthrodial joints are referred to as *synovial joints*. These joints facilitate locomotion in the musculoskeletal system. Synovial joints may be classified as *simple* or *compound*.

Simple synovial joints involve only two bones. They may be structured for flexion and extension only—hinge movement. Hinge joints (*ginglymoid*) have articular surfaces contoured to permit movement in a single plane and are supported by closely placed collateral ligaments that resist movement in other planes. The phalangeal joints are of this type. More flexible condyloid joints (*condyloarthrosis*) permit movement in more than a single plane—flexion, extension, abduction (turning outward or laterally), and adduction (turning inward or medially). Such joints present a contouring and ligamentous arrangement compatible with movement in different planes. The metacarpophalangeal articulation of the index finger is of this type. A still more flexible simple joint is the carpometacarpal joint of the thumb. Some synovial joints are structured to permit sliding movement between the united parts (*arthrodial*), the surfaces being flat or slightly curved and unrestrained by closely placed ligaments. Some joints have a ball and socket arrangement (*enarthrosis*), such as the hip joint.

Compound synovial joints involve three or more bones. When the sliding movement is quite limited, the term *amphiarthrosis* applies. This movement is seen in intercarpal, carpometacarpal, and intermetacarpal joints. Pivotal movement is termed *trochoid* and is seen in the elbow during pronation and supination of the forearm. Compound joints may be structured chiefly for hinge movement, such as the knee joint. Others have complete freedom of movement, such as the elbow joint, in which flexion, extension, abduction, adduction, and trochoid movement are possible.

Structural Characteristics of Synovial Joints

ENCAPSULATION.—The fibrous capsule is attached near the periphery of the articular surfaces. One can usually identify this attachment area on the dry bone, the surface thus enclosed being the nonvascularized pressure-bearing portion and indicative of the articular surface.

The capsule is well vascularized and innervated. The vessels supply the tissue fluid, which has free metabolic interchange with the synovial fluid within the joint cavity. The synovial membrane that secretes the synovial fluid lines the inner surface of the fibrous capsule and may overlie slightly the articular surfaces peripherally, especially if the articular body is convex. The synovial fluid supplies the nutritional and metabolic requirements of the nonvascularized tissues within the capsule. It also serves as joint lubricant and furnishes phagocytic capability. It fills the joint cavity. The capsule is innervated by sensory receptors for proprioceptive monitoring and conscious sensibility.

ARTICULAR SURFACES.—The articular surfaces of synovial joints are composed of a thin layer of hyaline cartilage which, except in the peripheral areas, is nonvascularized and noninnervated. This is referred to as *articular cartilage*.

LIMITATION OF JOINT MOVEMENTS.—The type, direction, and extent of movement of a joint during normal functioning is restricted by several factors:

1. Shape and structural relationship of the moving parts.
2. Size and location of the articular surfaces or facets.
3. Location and structure of the fibrous capsule.
4. Location, length, and structure of collateral ligaments.
5. Location and structure of other supporting articular ligaments.
6. Location and structure of check ligaments.
7. The stretching length of muscles that power the joint.
8. The presence of other structural restraints, such as surrounding tissues.

JOINT STABILITY AND MOVEMENT.—Normally, the articular surfaces of a synovial joint remain in sharp contact at all times. Separation of such articular surfaces constitutes luxation or dislocation. Sharp contact of the articular surfaces in the resting condition of the joint results from muscle tonus as modified by the effect of gravity. Positive gravitational force, as in weight-bearing joints, increases such contact. Negative gravitational effect, as for example in shoulder joints, stimulates the muscle spindles and reflexly increases muscle contraction, thus maintaining continuous sharp contact of the articular surfaces. Stability and movement are the product of muscle action, the type and range of useful movement being determined by integrated muscle activity, as limited by the structural factors that restrain joint movement (mentioned above). *All synovial joints are pressure-bearing joints.* It is the combination of simultaneous compression and movement that determines diarthrodial joint structure. The degree of pressure varies according to the demands of function.

MENISCUS.—A meniscus (from the Greek *meniskos,* meaning "crescent") is a wedge-shaped crescent of fibrocartilage or dense fibrous tissue, one side of which forms a marginal attachment at the articular capsule and the other two sides extend into the joint cavity and end in a free edge. The structure does not divide the joint cavity into separate compartments, nor does it restrict or confine the synovial fluid. It facilitates movements of the bony parts but does not act as a true articular surface, in that it is not a determinant of that movement. Two such structures are found in the knee joint, the medial meniscus attaching to the medial margin of the superior articular surface of the tibia and the lateral meniscus attaching to the lateral margin of the superior articular surface of the tibia.

SPECIAL FEATURES OF CRANIOMANDIBULAR ARTICULATION

The craniomandibular articulation consists of two synovial (true diarthrodial) joints, the right and left temporomandibular joints. These joints have characteristics that are not shared by all other synovial joints. It is essential that these special features be recognized and appreciated.

Phylogenic Heritage

Costen's syndrome included several symptoms, some clearly auricular, some temporomandibular. His therapy, which was unmistakably masticatory, seemed also to alleviate the auricular component of the complaint. Anatomists, however, insisted that the joint and ear symptoms be delineated, thus dividing the syndrome into two parts. Treatment of the ear portion remained to otolaryngologists, while treatment of the masticatory portion was allotted to dentists. It is interesting to note, however, that in due time researchers established an intimate structural relationship between the ear and the joint.

The mandibular joint of lower animal life has undergone considerable change, especially from the amphibia through the mammal-like reptiles (Fig 1–1).[2] In the mammal, the primitive jaw articulation of the lower ver-

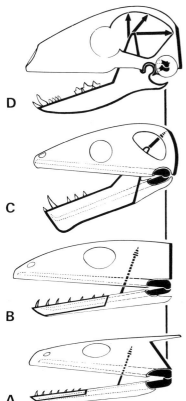

Fig 1–1.—Evolution of mammalian jaw joint. Back of skull and dentary bone in *heavy outline. Arrows* indicate muscle vectors. *A,* amphibian. Note notch on rear skull margin and muscle attached on undersurface of skull roof. *B,* reptile. Note increase in dentary bone and straight rear skull margin. *C,* mammal-like reptile. Note great increase in dentary bone with coronoid process and opening in skull roof (temporal fossa). *D,* mammal. Note dentary bone now contacts skull, forming the dentary-squamosal (temporomandibular) joint—an entirely new jaw joint. The primitive jaw articulation now forms the malleolar-incus joint of the ear ossicles. (From Du Brul E.L., in Sarnat B.G., Laskin D.M. (eds.): *The Temporomandibular Joint,* ed. 3, 1979. Courtesy of Charles C Thomas, Publisher, Springfield, Ill.)

tebrates is located in the middle ear as the articulation between the malleus and incus bones. The temporomandibular joint is phylogenically recent and peculiar to mammals.

In the important development of the craniomandibular articulation over eons of time, certain structures of the ear and temporomandibular joint became intimately related. The tensor tympani muscle, which flexes the tympanic membrane (arising from the cartilaginous portion of the eustachian tube and inserting into the malleus bone), is innervated by the mandibular division of the trigeminal nerve, which also innervates the masticatory muscles. Likewise, the tensor palati muscle, which elevates the palate and opens the eustachian tube by straightening it (arising from the sphenoid bone and wall of the eustachian tube and, after passing around the hamular process of the pterygoid bone, inserting into the aponeurosis of the soft palate), also is innervated by the mandibular division of the trigeminal nerve. Thus, the eustachian tube, which connects the cavity of the middle ear with the nasopharynx for the purpose of maintaining equalized air pressure on the ear drum, is under control of muscles innervated by nerves that subserve mastication. During deglutition, the palate is elevated to valve off the nasopharynx and the eustachian tubes are simultaneously opened. Thus, normal auditory function is intimately related to masticatory function. At the same time, the tensor tympani muscles also flex the ear drums, the sound of which may be heard accompanying the act of swallowing.

Another interesting structural relationship between the joint and the ear was brought to light by Pinto's discovery in 1962 of the mandibular-malleolar ligament.[9] This structure connects the temporomandibular capsule with the malleus bone, which in turn attaches to the tympanic membrane. Thus, when the condyle is translated forward, the ear drum is flexed. The sound of flexion can be heard by protruding the mandible or moving it laterally from side to side.

The structural and functional relationship between the masticatory apparatus and ears is intimate indeed, and symptoms in common should present no surprise or problem to dentists or otolaryngologists.

Chronological Changes in the Joint

The temporomandibular joint undergoes significant developmental change from infancy to skeletal maturity. These changes correspond to edentulousness at birth, eruption and articulation of the deciduous dentition, eruption and articulation of the permanent dentition, and skeletal maturation of the maxillary bones.

Although the joint at birth displays the structural components of the adult joint (Fig 1–2), it lies in line with the occlusal plane rather than an inch or more superior to it, as in the adult jaw (Fig 1–3). The articular eminence is low, the fossa is relatively flat, and hinge movement is the normal type of action. These features at birth are quite similar to the joints of carnivores. Throughout fetal life, the fibrous articular surfaces and interposing disc are vascularized and innervated. This state disappears as function induces compression of the disc between the condyle and temporal bone.[7] The growth changes that take place from birth to maturity are great.

The growth process is complex indeed and not completely understood. As the mandible moves forward and downward, its size increases in the opposite superior and posterior directions. This involves not only condylar growth, but also widespread remodeling of the entire bone, as resorptive and depository activity takes place. As the ramus grows posteriorly, the condyle simultaneously grows posteriorly and superiorly by active endochondral osseous proliferation. Intramembranous growth processes likewise take place throughout the osseous structures.

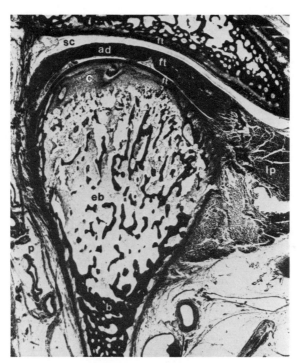

Fig 1–2.—The human temporomandibular joint at term. Note temporal bone *(t)*, superior compartment *(sc)* of the joint, the articular disc *(ad)*, cartilaginous area *(c)* of the condyle, endochondral bone *(eb)* formation, parotid gland *(p)*, and the lateral pterygoid muscle *(lp)*. The outer surfaces of the condyle and temporal portion of the joint cavity are covered with dense fibrous connective tissue *(ft)*. The articular disc is also composed of dense fibrous connective tissue. (From Furstman L., in Sarnat B.G., Laskin D.M. (eds.): *The Temporomandibular Joint,* ed. 3, 1979. Courtesy of Charles C Thomas, Publisher, Springfield, Ill.)

During the growth process, accommodation occurs first for the totally edentulous mouth, followed by eruption and final alignment of a complete deciduous dentition, spacing and shedding of deciduous teeth for succedaneous ones to follow, eruption and alignment of a complete adult dentition, and, finally, skeletal maturation and cessation of active developmental growth. Clinically, structural considerations of the temporomandibular joint at any particular time during the developmental years must take into account the state of development of the dentition at that time. The shape and size of the condyle relative to the depth of the articular fossa and elevation of the eminence should remain compatible as transition occurs from edentulous babyhood, through the relatively flat, end-to-end deciduous dentition, to the adult permanent dentition with its considerable interlock-

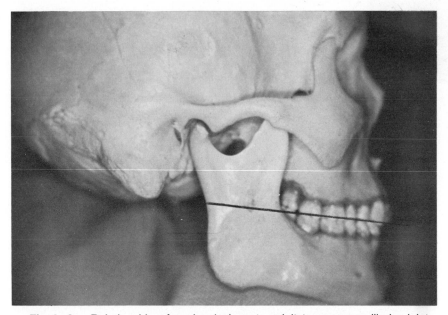

Fig 1–3.—Relationship of occlusal plane to adult temporomandibular joint. Note that mandibular condyle is an inch or more superior to plane of occlusion. At birth, it normally lies in line with plane of occlusion.

ing of occlusal surfaces. During certain transitional periods, change may be quite rapid. For example, in the critical transition from the deciduous to the permanent dentition (9 to 12 years of age, more or less), considerable increase in the height of the articular eminence may occur.

It should be noted that even after skeletal maturation and cessation of development, the process of osseous remodeling normally continues so that satisfactory accommodation in osseous structure can meet changing functional demands.

Bilaterality of the Craniomandibular Articulation

The craniomandibular articulation is bilateral, being composed of two joints, a left and a right temporomandibular joint, which form a functioning unit. They cannot function separately. What affects one joint must also influence the other.

Each of the two joints is compound and is classified as a ginglymo-arthrodial (hinge-sliding) joint. By definition, a compound joint involves three or more bones. In the temporomandibular joint, the articular disc functions as the third bone, supplying true articular surfaces above and below. Actually, the temporomandibular joint is a double joint composed of a lower ginglymoid and an upper arthrodial joint. Sicher described it as a hinge joint with a movable socket.[11]

It should be obvious that the articular disc is not a true meniscus, even though common usage justifies the term. Unfortunately, this misnomer has done much to foster confusion concerning the functioning of this joint, and it would be well to drop the term from use. The usual concept that the condyle articulates with the fossa-eminence, with an interposed meniscus, is not accurate. More correctly, the condyle articulates with the articular disc to form the disc-condyle complex, which in turn articulates with the temporal bone. The disc-condyle complex is a simple hinge joint. The upper joint is designed for sliding movement in any direction, the range being limited by structural restraints.

Articular Surfaces

The articular surfaces of the temporomandibular joints are different from other synovial joints (except those of the clavicles) in that they are not composed of hyaline cartilage. Rather, these surfaces are composed of non-vascularized and noninnervated *dense fibrous tissue* which functions like cartilage insofar as it is suited to the demands of movement and compression simultaneously.

This difference becomes important in the matter of regenerative capabilities of the joint. It is known that hyaline cartilage has low propensity in this regard when damaged or lost. The temporomandibular joints, however, enjoy a considerably greater potentiality—a feature of real importance in treatment planning. It is also known that degenerative arthritis is a primary disease of articular hyaline cartilage.[12] The temporomandibular joints do not have articular cartilage—an important departure from usual synovial joint structure.

Condylar Cartilage

Condylar cartilage is not articular cartilage. This distinction is important in the understanding of mandibular growth as well as of joint behavior. The condylar cartilage functions in the process of endochondral bone formation, differently, however, from epiphyseal cartilage in long bones. It is *growth cartilage*. In long bones the epiphyseal and articular cartilages are never confused because they are separated by bone tissue. In the mandibular condyle, however, the growth cartilage is on the surface of the bone just beneath the fibrous articular surface. Its location, no doubt, is the reason why it has so often been confused with true articular cartilage.

Condylar cartilage does not enter into the problems of joint function—

that is, sustaining compression and movement. Rather, it has to do with bone formation in the growth and development of the mandibular condyle. Deformity results when its function in growth is interfered with.

It is known that bone growth is intramembranous in tensile relationships and endochondral in compression relationships. The concept that endochondral growth pushes the bones apart has been questioned seriously. Presently, it is thought that displacement of osseous structures due to expansive effect of developing muscles and other soft tissues exerts tension on the tissues where the bones tend to move apart, thus triggering proliferation of bone and enlargement. Perhaps it is the location of compressive influence due to functional requirements (as with the mandibular condyle) that accounts for the presence of endochondrosis. It seems to be generally agreed that active remodeling at the articulation and, indeed, throughout the individual bone is an integral part of the process of growth and development.[4]

Remodeling

Remodeling involves morphologic changes in bone as an adaptive response to altered environmental demands. Structural adaptation of the articular surfaces of the temporomandibular joint is necessary for normal development of the craniofacial skeleton and for the changing demands of function of the masticatory system throughout life.

Remodeling is said to be *progressive* when proliferation of tissue occurs and *regressive* when osteoclastic resorption is evident. The extraosseous surface of the mandibular condyle is composed of three layers (Fig 1–4): a layer of nonvascularized dense fibrous tissue which constitutes the articular surface, a deeper zone of proliferative cells that can produce either a cartilaginous or an osseous matrix, and a still deeper layer of hyaline cartilage next to the bone. Remodeling is evidenced by increased activity in the proliferative zone. Early remodeling changes appear to be largely progressive, with thickening of the articular soft tissue taking place along with osseous change. Such change occurs more in the condylar than temporal surface, and little or none occurs in the articular disc.[6]

The degree of compressive stress seems to significantly influence changes within the stress-bearing portions of the joint. Moderate loading appears to facilitate normal remodeling. Excessive loading appears to arrest remodeling and may induce metaplasia of a hyaline cartilage–like tissue, not only in the articular surface of the condyle, but in the articular disc and upper articular surface as well. If compressive force is sufficiently great, localized resorption results.[8]

All such remodeling changes embrace an element of time. It takes time

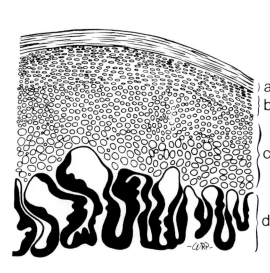

Fig 1–4.—The condylar cartilage has a fibrous covering *(a)* that overlies a region of rapidly proliferating prechondroblasts *(b)*. In area *c*, the cells have become chondrocytes that "mature" in the deeper part of the zone. Each cell undergoes hypertrophy, and a limited deposition of intercellular matrix occurs. Near zone *d*, the matrix calcifies, and cartilage resorption with subsequent bone deposition begins along the posterosuperior moving interface between *c* and *d*. (From Enlow D.H.: *Handbook of Facial Growth.* Philadelphia, W.B. Saunders Co., 1975. Reproduced with permission.)

for the biomechanical adaptations to occur. Adaptive changes, therefore, may be expected *if time permits*. If the demands for change are too rapid, however, degenerative breakdown may take place instead.

The temporomandibular joint is not a rigid, static, unchanging structure. Rather, like all other joints, it is adaptable to the demands of function, providing (1) the forces applied are not destructively excessive (such as movement of articular surfaces under sufficient pressure to induce frictional abuse), (2) the demands for change are not excessively rapid (such as acute trauma, too rapid orthodontic movement, or sudden changes due to natural or iatrogenic causes), and (3) the host conditions are not unsatisfactory for normal responsive behavior (such as age, illness, diabetes, and rheumatoid disease). It should be noted that the adaptive capability of the dentition far exceeds that of the joints. *Therefore, if therapeutic change is contemplated, it is better to attempt adaptation of the dentition to the joints rather than vice versa.*

Age should be considered in the biomechanical adaptive process of the joints. Clinically, the adaptive processes appear to be quite adequate during the developmental period and to remain so well into adult life. In later years, however, the obvious decrease in response suggests a serious decline in the adaptive and regenerative capability. This has bearing on treatment planning and prognosis.

Structural Requirements Imposed by Translatory Movement

The temporomandibular joint is the most complex of all synovial joints. The double-joint arrangement enables movements that are utter extremes. Hinge action in the lower joint is purely rotatory. Sliding action in the upper joint can take place in all directions, even pivotally. The extensive translatory movement of the disc-condyle complex gives the joint its great range of motion. This remarkable movement, which reaches a zenith in the higher primates, imposes, however, a number of structural requirements that should be well understood.

PROVISION FOR STABILITY.—Adequate stability during translation is necessary. Since the craniomandibular articulation functions bilaterally, the disc-condyle complexes are suspended bilaterally by two temporomandibular ligaments, one situated in the lateral portion of the articular capsule in each joint. These ligaments prevent dislocation inferiorly during the translatory cycle. They also limit posterior movement of the condyles, thus preventing posterior dislocation, especially at the end of a power stroke—even when edentulous.

Stability during the translatory cycle is maintained by firm contact between the disc-condyle complex and the eminence. This is accomplished by muscle action involving the posterior temporalis in combination with the inferior head of the lateral pterygoid muscle. During power strokes that force the teeth against a bolus of food, stability is ensured by action of the superior head of the lateral pterygoid muscle in two ways: (1) holding action applied to the condylar neck, thus permitting the return movement of the translatory cycle to be controlled until intercuspation takes place, and (2) firm anterior rotatory traction applied to the articular disc, thus drawing a thicker portion of disc firmly into the widened articular disc space created by torquing of the mandible.

During maximum intercuspation, stability is provided by the occlusion of the teeth themselves. This permits muscle action to drop back to the resting state as the dentition also assumes a position of physiologic rest.

CAPSULAR ATTACHMENT.—The temporomandibular articular capsule is attached to the condyle, disc, and temporal bone in such a manner as to create two separate joint cavities (with the help of the retrodiscal tissue), but not to interfere with or restrain the function of the condyle to translate anteriorly the full extent of the temporal articular surface. It attaches rather closely, therefore, in all but the posterior region of the joint, where it forms loose accordion-like folds. This permits the full translatory cycle to take place without capsular restraint as the folds open up.

RETRODISCAL TISSUE.—Since the articular disc is not a meniscus, but functions as an intervening bone with superior and inferior articular facets, *it is necessary that the two joint cavities be isolated so as to retain their separate portions of synovial fluid*. This separation is accomplished only partially by the disc itself. It is completed by the presence of a mass of loose connective tissue attached to the posterior edge of the articular disc and extending to and filling the loose folds of the posterior capsule. This tissue is well vascularized and innervated. Its upper and lower surface structures or laminae enter importantly into the functioning of the disc-condyle complex, as will be seen later. These surfaces are covered with synovial membrane. Therefore, the retrodiscal tissue is an important source of synovial fluid in both joint cavities.

As translation takes place, the loose, flexible retrodiscal tissue follows the disc-condyle complex. Thus, translatory movements are accomplished without compromising the integrity of the two joint cavities or the vascular structures that are the source of synovial fluid. This structural arrangement is unique and of great importance in the normal functioning of the joint.

Temporomandibular Kinematics

Like all synovial joints, the temporomandibular joints are under the control of the musculature with respect to proprioceptive and sensory guidance, habit patterns, and volition. Afferent monitoring input provides the CNS "computer" with a continuous inflow of signals arising from the oral mucosa, the mucogingival tissues, the muscular structures of the mouth, the periodontal ligaments, and the capsular and articular ligaments of the temporomandibular joints, as well as from the masticatory muscles themselves. This mass of sensory input helps guide the disc-condyle complex through the translatory cycles, each chewing movement being altered as needed by the particular demands of function at any particular moment. Deeply ingrained habit patterns become established so that chewing becomes unconscious and nearly automatic, unless volition is used to override habitual and muscle-guided movements.

When the teeth are out of contact, nondental sensory and proprioceptive signals dominate guidance of chewing movements. The periodontal receptors come into play as the teeth are stimulated by the contact of food and each other, thus modifying guidance by periodontal sensory input. It is important to understand, however, that another form of guidance that is not controlled by afferent input from any source or by volition becomes dominant as maximum intercuspation takes place. This is the effect of structural tooth form—the meshing of inclined planes of teeth—a force that is irresistible as the final determinant of joint position at the end of a

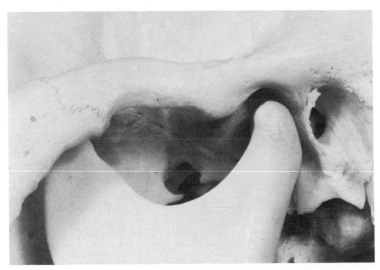

Fig 1–5.—Photograph of dry skull showing relationship of mandibular condyle to articular eminence with teeth in normal occlusion. No intervening articular disc is present. Note that occlusion of teeth prevents collapse of articular disc space.

chewing stroke or clenching the teeth. This force, which completely dominates the positioning of the condyle, occurs suddenly and every time the teeth are firmly occluded and disappears just as suddenly when the occluding effort is released.

Joint position is determined by muscle action (regardless of the factors of guidance and control) until the moment of maximum intercuspation, when a new and irresistible force suddenly determines that position. This new force lasts only as long as the teeth remain fully occluded. Unless strict harmony exists between these two factors that determine joint position, disruption of normal joint function may result. The tooth-dictated position must be harmonious with that determined by muscle action.

During maximum intercuspation, the fully occluded posterior teeth absorb most of the force exerted by the elevator muscles, thus relieving the joints and musculature of maintaining adequate stability. This may be witnessed by observing that the articular disc space does not collapse when the teeth are occluded in the absence of an interposed disc between condyle and articular eminence (Fig 1–5).

Temporomandibular joint kinematics, therefore, require strict harmony between the dentition and muscle action for normal functioning of the masticatory apparatus to take place. This is why temporomandibular disorders are a problem for clinical dentistry.

REFERENCES

1. Costen J.B.: Syndrome of ear and sinus symptoms dependent upon disturbed function of the temporomandibular joint. *Ann. Otol. Rhinol. Laryngol.* 43:1, 1934.
2. Du Brul E.L.: Evolution of the temporomandibular joint, in Sarnat B.G. (ed.): *The Temporomandibular Joint*, ed. 2. Springfield, Ill., Charles C Thomas, Publisher, 1964, pp. 3–27.
3. Du Brul E.L.: *Sicher's Oral Anatomy*, ed. 7. St. Louis, C.V. Mosby Co., 1980.
4. Enlow D.H.: The condyle and facial growth, in Sarnat B.G., Laskin D.M. (eds.): *The Temporomandibular Joint*, ed. 3. Springfield, Ill., Charles C Thomas, Publisher, 1979, pp. 70–84.
5. Krogh-Poulsen A.W., Moelhave A.: Om discus articularis temporomandibularis. *Tondlaegebladt* 61:265, 1957.
6. Hansson T.: Temporomandibular joint changes related to dental occlusion, in Solberg W.K., Clark G.T. (eds.): *Temporomandibular Joint Problems.* Chicago, Quintessence Publishing Co., 1980, pp. 129–143.
7. Levy B.M.: Embryological development of the temporomandibular joint, in Sarnat B.G. (ed.): *The Temporomandibular Joint*, ed. 2. Springfield, Ill., Charles C Thomas, Publisher, 1964, pp. 59–70.
8. Meikle M.C.: Remodeling, in Sarnat B.G., Laskin D.M.: (eds.): *The Temporomandibular Joint*, ed. 3. Springfield, Ill., Charles C Thomas, Publisher, 1979, pp. 205–226.
9. Pinto O.F.: A new structure related to the TM joint and middle ear. *J. Prosthet. Dent.* 12:95, 1962.
10. Rees L.A.: The structure and function of the temporomandibular joint. *Br. Dent. J.* 96:125, 1954.
11. Sicher H.: *Oral Anatomy.* St. Louis, C.V. Mosby Co., 1949.
12. Toller P.A.: Temporomandibular arthropathy. *Proc. R. Soc. Med.* 67:153, 1974.

2 / Structural Components of the Craniomandibular Articulation

A GOOD UNDERSTANDING of the functional anatomy of the craniomandibular articulation is an absolute prerequisite for accurate diagnosis and effective treatment of temporomandibular disorders, and necessarily is the basis for judging when departures from normal occur.

THE CHEWING UNIT

The process of mastication requires a complete functioning unit, structurally interrelated and biologically integrated. Chewing is a mechanical process in which physical laws cannot be ignored. Laws governing movement, force, resistance, friction, and noise must be given due consideration. Like locomotion, mastication involves structures of the musculoskeletal system that behave according to certain principles of biomechanics.

The chief working component of the mouth proper, relative to mastication, is the dentition—teeth functioning in such a way as to hold, incise, tear, and grind foods. The lips, cheeks, tongue, and palate position and control the foods in the mouth. These structures are muscle-activated and neurologically guided by central direction, reflex activities, and feedback mechanisms. The teeth are anchored in bony frameworks that are bilaterally connected by the craniomandibular articulation, which is composed of two separate but functionally related temporomandibular joints. Skeletal muscles power the mandibular frame. They are activated and guided by impulses from the CNS in response to preconditioned habit patterns, reflex activity, feedback mechanisms, and volition. Swallowing invokes activity of the tongue, palate, pharynx, epiglottis, and esophagus. Saliva is an essential factor in mastication; it softens and binds food particles, initiates the digestive process, lubricates the oral structures, and facilitates swallowing. Salivation is a glandular activity under control of the visceral nervous system and responsive to systemic factors. To all this is added an effective sensory system for detecting and selectively choosing proper foods. Influencing the whole process are the factors of systemic relationships, emotional situations, and volition.

Mastication involves many structures—bones, joints, muscles, teeth, glands, nerves of different types, blood vessels—and systemic and central nervous system processes. Any attempt to examine one part in isolation from the rest is futile. Since the objective of this book is to consider particularly temporomandibular disorders, only the craniomandibular articulation and its activating musculature will be taken into account. This is not to imply that other structures of the chewing unit, particularly the occlusion of teeth, are any less important. Each is essential in its own way to the normal functioning of the whole system.

Craniomandibular Articulation

In man, the articulation of a one-piece mandible with the cranium is a bilateral structure joining the mandibular condyles with articular facets on the temporal bone, the right and left temporomandibular joints. All movements of the mandible affect both joints. Functionally, they cannot be considered as isolated structures.

These joints are compression-movement articulations, which requires that the pressure-bearing articular surfaces be nonvascularized and noninnervated. As such, they are classified as diarthrodial or synovial joints.

Each temporomandibular joint is capable of two distinct movements, rotating and sliding. Rotation or hinge action is confined strictly to the condyle-articular disc portion of the joint, while sliding movement is confined strictly to the articular disc-temporal bone portion. The temporomandibular joint functions as a *compound joint,* which by definition requires the presence of at least three bones. The articular disc, therefore, functions as the third bone interposed between the condyle and temporal bone. The inferior surface of the disc is a true articular facet that articulates with a similar facet on the mandibular condyle. The superior surface of the disc is also a true articular facet that articulates with a similar but much larger facet on the temporal bone. Thus, the temporomandibular joint is a true compound joint—really a double joint, one above the other. It is a lower hinge joint and an upper sliding joint, all in a single capsule. As such, it is classified as a ginglymo-arthrodial joint.

The two joints that constitute the temporomandibular joint have several structures in common, namely:

1. The *articular disc together with the retrodiscal tissue,* which separates the temporomandibular joint into two distinct joints.

2. The *capsular ligament,* which encapsulates separately the two joints, thus confining the synovial fluid to separate compartments or synovial cavities.

3. The *musculature,* which provides for stability and movement in both joints.

ARTICULAR CAPSULE

The capsular ligament is composed of fibrous connective tissue. It attaches to the periphery of the articular facets on the temporal bone above and the mandibular condyle below. The sides of the capsule anteriorly are little more than loose connective tissue supporting the synovial membrane. The temporomandibular ligament strongly reinforces the lateral wall of the capsule. Anteriorly, the capsule fuses with the articular disc. Posteriorly, it attaches to the retrodiscal tissue in accordion-like folds that permit freedom of movement of the disc-condyle complex anteriorly.

The capsule offers little restraint on mandibular movements except in the outer ranges. Rather, it appears to relate more to the dynamics of synovial fluid. In the closed position, the fluid in both upper and lower joint cavities appears to be distributed evenly anterior and posterior to the disc. In forward translation, much of the fluid is located posteriorly, the synovial fluid conforming to the shape of the capsule. This suggests that functioning of the capsule is an important factor in lubricating and nourishing the articular surfaces, the fluid being swished back and forth between the articulating surfaces as translatory movements take place.

The fibrous capsule is well vascularized and innervated. It is lined with synovial membrane which secretes the synovial fluid into the joint cavities. The vascular supply is chiefly from the superficial temporal artery.

Afferent nerve fibers for proprioception and general sensibility are branches of the auriculotemporal, masseteric, and posterior deep temporal nerves.[4] Fibers of the auriculotemporal innervate the posterior capsule and retrodiscal tissue; those of the masseteric and temporal nerves innervate the anterior part of the capsular ligament. These nerves terminate in the periphery of the articular disc. Free nerve endings, generally conceded to mediate pain sensation, are abundant throughout the capsule, thus giving it the propensity to sense pain. Ruffini's corpuscles, Golgi tendon organs, and Pacinian corpuscles are found in the capsular ligament, especially in the lateral and posterolateral parts, thus proprioceptively monitoring condylar position and movement. Visceral fibers, accompanying somatic fibers of the auriculotemporal nerve, supply the blood vessels of the capsule.[2]

DISC-CONDYLE COMPLEX

The articulation of the mandibular condyle with the articular disc forms a simple hinge joint (ginglymoid), which henceforth will be referred to as the *disc-condyle complex*.

Articular Surfaces

The articular facet of the mandibular condyle is small compared with that of the temporal bone (Fig 2–1). It is rounded mediolaterally and quite convex anteroposteriorly. The posterior margin of the articular surface extends a considerable distance, permitting more extensive rotation of the disc posteriorly than anteriorly. The articular surface is composed of dense, nonvascularized, noninnervated fibrous tissue rather than cartilage, as in most other synovial joints. This tissue is quite thin over most of the articular facet but thickens appreciably in the anterosuperior aspect, indicating the area best suited to sustain maximum pressure. A few cartilaginous cells may be seen, especially in higher age periods.

Immediately beneath the dense fibrous articular surface is the *proliferative zone*, the cells of which have the potentiality to produce either a cartilaginous or osseous matrix. Deeper to the proliferative zone and adjacent to the osseous structure of the condyle is the *condylar cartilage* (see Fig 1–4). It should be understood that this pertains to endochondral growth, which in some respects simulates epiphyseal cartilage of long bones. It is distinctively different structurally and functionally from articular cartilage of other synovial joints and should not be confused with it.

The inferior surface of the articular disc forms the other facet that artic-

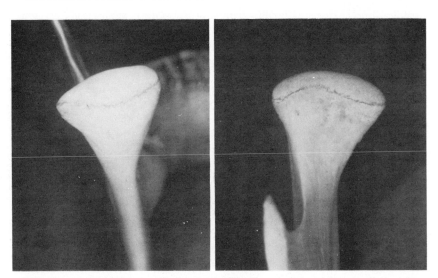

Fig 2–1.—Subarticular bone of mandibular condyle. *Left,* posterior view. *Right,* anterior view. Attachment of capsular ligament outlined with pencil. Note that articular facet is more extensive posteriorly.

ulates with the condyle to make up the disc-condyle complex. This surface is slightly concave mediolaterally and boldly concave anteroposteriorly, making it compatible with the condylar surface for flexion-extension movement in the sagittal plane.

The shape of the articular surfaces permits freedom of hinge movement between the disc and condyle anteroposteriorly.

Articular Disc

The articular disc is composed of dense fibrous tissue that is nonvascular and noninnervated except in the peripheral areas. A few cartilaginous cells may be seen, especially in higher age periods. The size and shape of the disc are determined by the size and contour of its lower and upper surfaces, which are determined by the shape of the condylar and temporal facets, respectively. The articular disc is thinner in its central portion. The much thicker posterior border relates to the angulation of the articular eminence: *the steeper this angulation, the thicker the posterior margin of disc*.

The superior surface of the disc is flattened and slightly concave anteroposteriorly. It is compatible with the fossa-eminence articular surface for sliding movements.

The articular disc is moderately flexible, so that it is adaptable to the osseous-supported articular facets during translatory movements. It is not compressible, however, to an extent that is radiographically apparent.

Discal Ligaments

Collateral ligaments attaching the articular disc to the medial and lateral poles of the condyle were described by Krogh-Poulsen and Moelhave in 1957.[3] These nonelastic structures, like other true ligaments, are composed of collagenous connective tissue fibers. *They do not stretch*. If subjected to abusive and repeated strain, they may elongate, thus impairing their efficiency to passively restrain discal movement. Like all collateral ligaments, these ligaments serve to restrict the movements of the joint to hinge action in a single plane. Being short and closely placed to the articulating surfaces, the ligaments limit gross movement between the articular disc and mandibular condyle to rotation. They are not so rigidly attached, however, as to prevent slight shifting movements of the disc laterally. The discal ligaments attach the articular disc to the condyle in such a manner as to cause it to passively follow the condyle wherever it moves. They resist displacement between disc and condyle. *The disc may rotate forward (prolapse) on the condyle, but it cannot be bodily displaced anteriorly or posteriorly as long as these ligaments are intact and functional*.

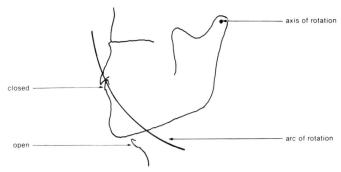

Fig 2–2.—Tracing from lateral radiographs of face in *closed* and *open* positions. Condylar *axis of rotation* is indicated at about center of condyle. An arc from axis of rotation drawn through the incisal edge of mandibular incisor in closed position describes the *arc of rotation*. Note that in normal translatory opening the position of mandibular incisor is anterior to arc of rotation.

The discal ligaments are vascularized and innervated. When strained, they may sense pain. When injured, they may become inflamed. They proprioceptively monitor position and movement.

Like all hinge joints, the disc-condyle complex has an anatomical axis of rotation. It passes mediolaterally through the attachments of the articular disc to the condyle: that is, through the medial and lateral condylar poles. If projected onto the face, this axis terminates at a point near the center of the mandibular condyle. If projected medially, it crosses its fellow of the opposite side near the anterior margin of the foramen magnum. Since the disc-condyle complex moves anteroposteriorly during translatory movements, the intercondylar hinge axis also moves. To be a useful point of orientation on the face, the intercondylar hinge axis registration should be accomplished by using rotatory movement of the condyle only. The degree to which translation is permitted, therefore, represents technical error.

The arc of rotation of the disc-condyle complex is the arc of a circle, the radius of which extends from the anatomical rotatory axis of the condyle. If this radius is projected to the mandibular incisor area, a circle is described, a segment of which represents the arc of rotation at the incisor area. It should be noted that normal translatory opening follows a path that terminates anterior to this arc of rotation (Fig 2–2).

Retrodiscal Tissue

The retrodiscal tissue attaches to the posterior edge of the articular disc. It extends posteriorly to and fuses with the loose, folded, accordion-like articular capsule. Its *superior lamina* attaches to the tympanic plate. Composed of connective tissue containing many elastic fibers, this lamina has the quality of elasticity by which it is able to counteract the forward traction of the superior lateral pterygoid muscle on the articular disc. Except during full forward translation, when this superior lamina is stretched, the effect of muscle tonus in the superior lateral pterygoid muscle is dominant and exceeds the elastic traction of the retrodiscal tissue. *Therefore, the articular disc normally occupies the most forward rotated position on the condyle that is permitted by the width of the articular disc space.* This mechanism supplies a high degree of stability to the joint by maintaining sharp contact between the articulating parts at all times.

The *inferior retrodiscal lamina* attaches anteriorly to the articular disc and posteriorly just below the posterior margin of the condylar articular facet. It is different from the superior lamina in that it is composed chiefly of collagenous fibers, making it nonelastic. This lamina serves as a check ligament that passively limits forward rotation of the disc on the condyle. Like all ligaments, it does not enter actively into disc functioning.

The *body of retrodiscal tissue* consists of loose connective tissue that is highly vascularized and innervated. Synovial membrane covers both the superior and inferior laminae. Thus, the retrodiscal tissue is a major contributor to synovial fluid metabolism, which is essential to the normal functioning of a synovial joint. It ensures free metabolic exchange, nutrition, and lubrication of the articulating surfaces in both upper and lower joints, whether at rest or during translatory movement. Sensory elements of the auriculotemporal nerve furnish receptors for proprioceptive monitoring of position and movement, as well as sensibility to pain.

ARTICULATION OF DISC-CONDYLE COMPLEX WITH TEMPORAL BONE

The upper part of the compound temporomandibular joint consists of the disc-condyle complex articulating with the articular facet of the temporal bone in a manner that permits freedom of sliding (arthrodial) movement. This requires flattened articular surfaces that are not restrained by ligamentous structures.

Fossa-Eminence Articular Surface

The temporal articular facet that accommodates the disc-condyle complex occupies the anterolateral part of the glenoid fossa and the whole of the articular eminence (Fig 2–3). As indicated by evidence of attachment of the capsular ligament on the dry bone, the articular surface falls safely clear of adjacent bony structures. Laterally, the articular surface ends sev-

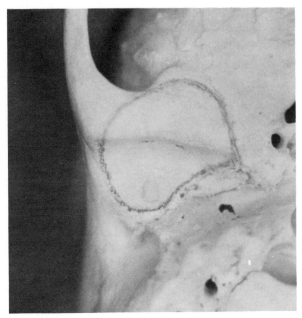

Fig 2–3.—Subarticular bone of temporal articular facet. Attachment of capsular ligament is outlined with pencil. Articular surface is narrow posteriorly, widest at articular eminence. Structures medial and posterior are not included within capsular attachment. Note forward extent of articular surface.

eral millimeters short of the outer margin of the inferior surface of the supra-articular crest.

Since lateral flat-plate radiographs of the temporomandibular joint cause this outer margin to obscure the true articular surface of the temporal bone, what appears as the upper osseous surface is obviously an artifact (Fig 2–4). This discrepancy increases proportionately in the eminence region as the distance of the articular facet from the edge of the supra-articular crest becomes greater. The true osseous surface, which lies slightly medially and superiorly, is visualized radiographically only by the tomographic method. *Thus, the inclination of the articular eminence is not as steep as it appears to be on flat-plate radiography, and the true articular disc space is wider than is radiographically apparent.*

The supra-articular crest anterior to the articular eminence bows out to form the zygomatic arch, thus obscuring the osseous joint surface anterior to the eminence. The shape of the articular surface anterior to the crest of the articular eminence is a gentle slope superiorly, being nearly flat in

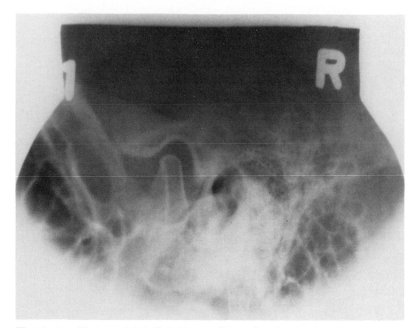

Fig 2–4.—Transparietal flat-plate radiograph of temporomandibular joint. Note that what appears to be subarticular osseous structure is actually the more dense outer margin of the joint; what appears to be articular eminence is articular tubercle. The anterior slope of articular eminence is obscured by the zygomatic arch.

many joints (Fig 2–5). It does not follow the dramatic upward sweep of the lateral margin of the articular tubercle, as visualized radiographically.

Mediolaterally, the temporal articular facet is gently concave throughout its full anteroposterior sweep. It conforms to the slight mediolateral convexity of the articular facet of the mandibular condyle. Thus, the articular disc is of fairly uniform thickness mediolaterally, being gently concave below and convex above.

The extreme anterior and posterior borders of the temporal articular surface lie nearly parallel to the Frankfurt horizontal plane (Fig 2–6). Between these extremities, the upward concavity of the fossa just about equals the downward convexity in the eminence area. Since the shadow of the *superior margin* of the supra-articular crest is visible radiographically, and since this structure *in the eminence area* is nearly parallel to the Frankfurt plane, a useful means of estimating the inclination of the articular eminence is radiographically available (Fig 2–7). It should be noted, however, that the actual osseous surface is a few degrees flatter than this would indicate.

The articular surface proper of the temporal facet, like the condylar facet

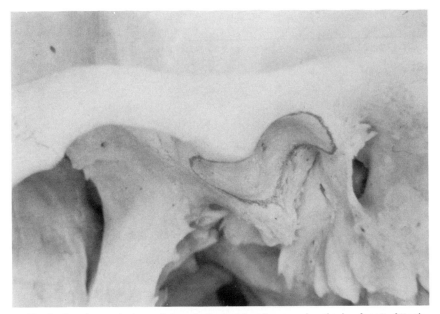

Fig 2–5.—Lateral view of dry skull showing temporal articular facet. Attachment of capsular ligament is outlined with pencil. Note that anterior slope of articular eminence is only moderately inclined superiorly compared with the posterior slope.

below, is composed of a thin layer of nonvascularized, noninnervated, dense fibrous tissue. Over the posterior surface of the articular eminence, this tissue thickens perceptibly, indicating the area best suited to sustain maximum pressure. Anatomically, the direction of greatest pressure from the mandible to the temporal bone is upward and forward. It projects from the anteriorly inclined mandibular condyle, through the thin central portion of disc, and into the body of the articular eminence, which is massively braced.

Beneath the fibrous articular surface is a proliferative zone of cells that function in the same manner as in the condyle. The occasional presence of a hyaline cartilage-like proliferation in the temporal articular surface only demonstrates the potential of the cells of the proliferative zone to differentiate into a cartilaginous matrix.

Disc-Condyle Complex Articular Surface

The disc-condyle complex articulates with the temporal bone to form the upper sliding portion of the temporomandibular joint. The superior surface of the articular disc is the lower articular surface of this sliding joint. The

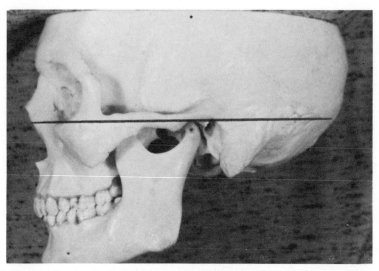

Fig 2–6.—Dry skull with Frankfurt horizontal indicated. Note that superior surface of supra-articular crest in the area of the articular eminence is nearly parallel to the Frankfurt plane. Since the supra-articular crest is clearly visible on a flat-plate radiograph of the temporomandibular joint, it serves as an accurate means of estimating the angle of inclination of the articular eminence.

surface is shaped to be compatible with the fossa-eminence articular facet. Mediolaterally, it is slightly convex. Anteroposteriorly, it is slightly concave. The contour of this surface correlates with the prominence of the articular eminence. The flatness and compatibility of the articular surfaces, the absence of collateral ligaments, and the loose attachment of the capsular ligament ensure freedom of sliding movement in all directions. The slight mediolateral convexity of the disc, with compatible concavity of the temporal facet, strongly favors sliding movement in the sagittal plane.

Temporomandibular Ligament Suspension

The mandible, more particularly the pair of disc-condyle complexes, is suspended from the craniofacial skeleton by two strong *lateral ligaments,* currently referred to by anatomists under the older terminology, *the temporomandibular ligaments.*[1] Although bilateral, as related to the whole craniomandibular articulation, these ligaments do not function as collateral ligaments. By definition, collateral ligaments are paired to a single joint for the specific purpose of restricting extension and flexion to one plane only. The temporomandibular ligaments serve quite a different purpose. They are the suspensory mechanism of the mandible that resists downward and posterior displacement. As such, they protect the individual temporomandibular joint against gross disarticulation inferiorly and posteriorly.

The temporomandibular ligament is composed of two parts: an *outer oblique portion*, arising from the outer surface of the articular tubercle and extending down and back to insert into the outer surface of the condylar neck, and an *inner horizontal portion*, arising from the same area and running horizontally backward to insert into the lateral pole of the condyle and posterior part of the articular disc (Fig 2–8).[1]

The temporomandibular ligament is in close structural relationship with the lateral aspect of the capsular ligament, which it strongly reinforces. Its attachments are in intimate structural relationship with the lateral discal ligament. The outer oblique portion attaches to the condyle below the lateral pole; the inner horizontal portion attaches to the lateral condylar pole. The intimate arrangement of these important structures has special significance in some traumatic conditions of the temporomandibular joint. For example, a torn capsule, in itself, has only minor significance: that of pos-

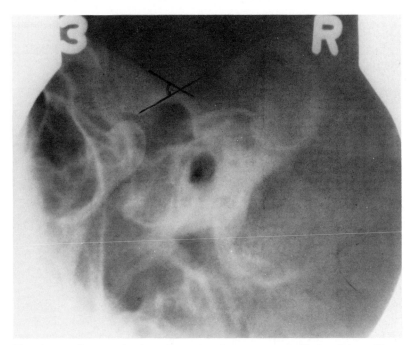

Fig 2–7.—Transparietal radiograph of temporomandibular joint. Observe shadow of supra-articular crest. Angle formed by supra-articular crest and posterior slope of articular eminence indicates the approximate angle of inclination of the eminence in degrees. Average inclination is 30 to 60 degrees. This eminence is about 57 degrees.

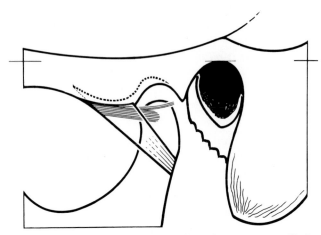

Fig 2–8.—Diagram of adaptive construction of temporomandibular ligament. Condyle is pulled out of position and disc is omitted for clarity. Outline of articular eminence (surface) is represented by heavy interrupted line. Outer, oblique band runs from articular tubercle to condylar neck. Inner, horizontal band *(hatched)* runs from the articular tubercle to the lateral condylar pole and back of disc. (From Du Brul E.L.: *Sicher's Oral Anatomy,* ed. 7. St. Louis, C.V. Mosby Co., 1980. Reproduced with permission.)

sible fibrotic contracture due to cicatrization which could reduce condylar movement in the outer ranges. Such a torn capsule, however, could seriously disrupt normal disc-condyle complex functioning by detaching the lateral discal ligament. Or it could alter the protective suspensory mechanism by rupturing one or both portions of the temporomandibular ligament. Such minor trauma could have major consequences. Likewise, surgical opening of the articular capsule cannot be done with impunity, since it is fraught with similar consequences.

The outer oblique portion of the temporomandibular ligament protects against excessive dropping of the mandibular condyle during translatory movements. It imposes, therefore, a lower suspensory limit and so determines the extreme lower range of movement for the intercondylar hinge axis.

The inner horizontal portion limits how far the disc-condyle complex can go posteriorly. Normally this limit is not reached because intercuspation of teeth at the end of a power stroke firmly anchors the condylar position. In posterior edentulousness, however, the final determinant of condylar position depends on the holding action of the lateral pterygoid muscle, with the limit to posterior movement being established by the temporomandibular ligament. A serious consequence of inadequate posterior dental support is sequential elongation of this ligament until it no longer restrains the condyle from damaging the structures posterior to the articular disc. It should be understood that these ligamentous structures (discal ligaments, capsular ligament, and temporomandibular ligament) are innervated for proprioceptive monitoring of movement and position. Under strain, various effects may tend to disrupt normal muscle action. These ligaments also are innervated for pain detection and are vascularized. Thus, inflammatory processes may develop if injury is sustained.

The inner horizontal portion of the temporomandibular ligament has a special restraining function: it arrests posterior condylar movement during pivoting of the working joint when lateral excursions are made. It serves two important purposes: (1) it prevents encroachment of the pivoting lateral pole of the condyle on structures posterior to it, and (2) it holds condyle and disc in their normal relationship during the pivoting (trochoid) movement, thus reducing strain on the discal ligaments. It is this restraining influence on the lateral pole of the condyle that alters mandibular movement and causes the condyle to rotate vertically around the lateral pole rather than around the anatomical vertical axis.

Translatory Cycle

The temporomandibular joint is structured to deliver two movements, namely, hinge or rotatory movement in the disc-condyle complex and sliding or translatory movement between the disc-condyle complex and the temporal bone. The translatory cycle is a combination of these two movements.

JOINT STABILITY.—Empty-mouth movements constitute the bulk of temporomandibular functions. Empty-mouth movements include all activities except those which involve special contraction of elevator muscles, such as chewing movements or special use of the jaws for holding objects. Empty-mouth functioning goes on 24 hours a day—an example is swallowing.

During empty-mouth translatory cycles, stability is maintained by continuous sharp contact of the articulating parts. This is accomplished by muscle tonus as affected by gravity. The weight of the mandible represents negative gravitational force that stimulates the muscle spindles in elevator masticatory muscles, thereby initiating the myotatic or stretch reflex and automatically increasing tonicity in those muscles. The posterior fibers of the temporalis and the inferior head of the lateral pterygoid muscle are of particular importance in the maintenance of continuous sharp contact during translatory movements.

Chewing brings into play power strokes, which impose a special burden on the musculature to maintain adequate stability. Such strokes have a marked effect on interarticular pressure in both the chewing side and the opposite joint. The articular disc, in response to contraction of the superior head of the lateral pterygoid muscle, plays a decisive role in maintaining sharp contact of the articulating parts during the entire power stroke until intercuspation of the teeth takes over at the end of the stroke.

RESTRICTION OF MOVEMENTS.—The gross extent of jaw opening is limited by such extra-articular influences as the stretching length of the elevator muscles and the size of the orifice of the mouth. The capsular ligament offers little resistance to movement. Only the posterior portion tends to limit anterior movement of the condyle.

Within the joint, rotatory movement of the disc on the condyle is limited anteriorly by the inferior retrodiscal lamina and posteriorly by the anterior capsular ligament. Violation of hinge movement and separation between disc and condyle are resisted by the discal lateral ligaments. At the end of power strokes and during pivoting movements, the temporomandibular ligament imposes limitation on movement. Gross dislocation between temporal bone and disc-condyle complex is resisted by the temporomandibular ligament posteriorly and inferiorly.

ACTIVATORS OF MOVEMENT.—The masticatory muscles constitute the source of power for movement of the mandible. The mouth is opened by depressor action of the digastric and mylohyoid muscles in conjunction with contraction of the inferior head of the lateral pterygoid muscles. This activity is best demonstrated when the mouth is opened against resistance. When there is no resistance to opening, very little active muscle contraction is required to overcome the effect of muscle tonus in the elevator muscles. Closing the mouth is accomplished by contraction of the elevator muscles. Empty-mouth closure requires minimal muscular effort. Power strokes require strong contraction of elevator muscles, controlled by a holding action exerted by the depressor and the lateral pterygoid muscles. Protrusion and lateral excursion are executed by contraction of the inferior head of the lateral pterygoid muscles bilaterally and unilaterally, respectively. Retrusion of the mandible from the forward translated position is activated by contraction of posterior fibers of the temporalis and deep portion of the masseter in conjunction with the mylohyoid and digastric muscles. With all such movements, the activators are resisted by antagonists that exert holding and controlling effects. Active movement, therefore, invokes some degree of muscle activity from antagonist muscles as well.

Mandibular movements are accomplished by the complex interaction of many muscles, the usefulness of which requires a high degree of muscular coordination. Jaw movements are learned over a considerable period of time. Unconscious mandibular activity is guided largely by preconditioned habit patterns that become deeply ingrained and tend to resist change. Volitional movements, however, easily override such habitual muscle action. The product of conscious voluntary mandibular movement may or may not conform to habitual chewing movements and, therefore, may or may not be compatible with normal joint functioning. The immediate guidance of muscle action on an automatic level is the product of afferent input from oral tissues, periodontal ligaments, articular ligaments, and the muscles themselves.

The final determinant of joint position is tooth form, the result of intercuspation of teeth. Normal functioning depends on a high degree of harmony between the forces imposed by the action of muscles and those of the occluded dentition.

THE CYCLE.—The translatory cycle is a combination of rotatory and translatory movement. It begins from a rest position that is determined by muscle tonus, when the musculature is in a state of physiologic rest. The forward phase of the cycle consists of the disc-condyle complex moving downward and forward along the posterior slope of the articular eminence. It rounds the crest of the eminence and then moves forward along the articular plane that forms the anterior surface of the articular eminence. The return phase of the translatory cycle is a retracing of the disc-condyle complex back to rest position. Empty-mouth movements accomplish the translatory cycle with minimal interarticular pressure, but enough to maintain continuous sharp contact of the articulating parts. The translatory cycle is similar, whether it occurs with protrusion, lateral excursion, or opening. The difference lies in the degree of rotation mixed with translation, and whether the cycle is bilateral or unilateral. When the translatory cycle is unilateral (as in the balancing joint during a lateral excursion), the disc-condyle complex moves medially as it descends the articular eminence. This displaces the complex slightly in an inferior direction as the outer limit of lateral excursion is reached. Simultaneously, the opposite (working side) disc-condyle complex pivots until the inner horizontal portion of the temporomandibular ligament arrests further posterior movement of the lateral pole. From that point on, the disc-condyle complex rotates around a vertical axis that passes through the lateral pole rather than the center of the condyle. Ordinarily, the forces of tooth form initiated by intercuspation of teeth do not influence the translatory cycle during empty-mouth movements.

Power strokes alter the translatory cycle considerably in the return phase. Such cycle begins from rest position. It goes through the forward phase and begins the return phase, as described, until the bolus of food is encountered. As power is brought to bear on the food object, torquing of the mandible takes place. This alters the interarticular pressure in both joints. It continues to exert influence until the teeth penetrate the food object and come into full occlusion. Afferent input guidance changes during the power stroke as periodontal receptors are stimulated. The power stroke ends with maximum intercuspation, followed by relaxation of the musculature to the rest position. This brings into play the dominant positioning force of tooth form as maximum intercuspation is achieved. The dominating influence of tooth form ceases as biting is released and the muscles relax. The final determinant of joint position exerted by firmly occluded inclined planes of the teeth may or may not be compatible with the position established by muscle action alone.

It should be evident that the effect of the dentition on the translatory cycle occurs with power strokes. This stimulates the periodontal receptors, thus influencing muscle guidance. It initiates the element of tooth form—the final determinant of joint position as maximum intercuspation begins and ends. It should also be noted that empty-mouth clenching of teeth (bruxism), with or without movement, brings similar forces into play that have considerable influence on the temporomandibular joints and the musculature.

REFERENCES

1. Du Brul E.L.: *Sicher's Oral Anatomy*, ed. 7. St. Louis, C.V. Mosby Co., 1980.
2. Kawamura Y.: Neurophysiology, in Sarnat B.G., Laskin D.M. (eds.): *The Temporomandibular Joint*, ed. 3. Springfield, Ill., Charles C Thomas, Publisher, 1979, pp. 114–126.
3. Krogh-Poulsen A.W., Moelhave A.: Om discus articularis temporomandibularis. *Tondlaegebladt* 61:265, 1957.
4. Thilander B.: Innervation of the temporomandibular joint capsule in man. *Trans. R. School Dent.* 7:1, 1961.

3 / Biomechanics of the Temporomandibular Joint

THE ARTICULAR DISC of the temporomandibular joint is an integral part of a compound joint, the two parts of which move in quite different ways. The performance of its duties entails intricate functional movements that need to be understood well. The biomechanics of the temporomandibular joint are determined by the morphology and structural arrangement of its parts (Fig 3–1).

ARTICULAR DISC AS A COMPONENT OF TWO JOINTS

The disc-condyle complex is a simple hinge joint, complete in every detail. The shape of the articular facets of the mandibular condyle and lower surface of articular disc is compatible for rotatory hinge action in the sagittal plane. These articular surfaces are supported laterally by strong, closely placed, collateral ligaments that attach the disc to the medial and lateral poles of the condyle. The complex is encapsulated by the capsular ligament. The retrodiscal tissue completes the isolation of the synovial cavity and supplies vital synovial fluid. The inferior retrodiscal lamina acts as a check ligament to limit forward rotation of the disc on the condyle.

The disc-condyle complex, in turn, moves bodily in a sliding manner along the glenoid fossa and articular eminence of the temporal bone. It forms a sliding joint that is complete in every detail. The shape of the articular facets on the temporal bone and superior surface of the articular disc is compatible with sliding movement in all directions, but favors movement in the sagittal plane. These sliding joints are suspended by two strong temporomandibular ligaments in a manner that limits inferior and posterior displacement of the disc-condyle complexes. However, they do not restrict surface-contact sliding movement in either of the temporomandibular joints. The upper sliding joint is loosely encapsulated by the capsular ligament. The retrodiscal tissue completes the isolation of the upper synovial cavity, supplies vital synovial fluid, and facilitates extensive anteroposterior sliding movement of the disc-condyle complex. The superior lamina stabilizes the rotatory position of the disc on the condyle by counteracting the forward pull of the superior head of the lateral pterygoid muscle. It does

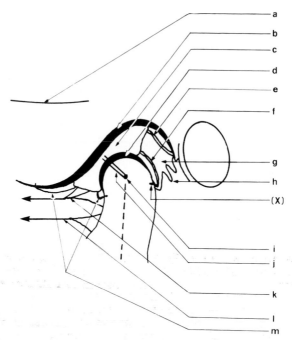

Fig 3–1.—Schematic drawing illustrates essential structures that constitute the functioning temporomandibular joint: *a*, supra-articular crest; *b*, temporal articular surface, composed of nonvascular fibrous tissue; *c*, articular disc; *d*, condylar articular surface, composed of nonvascular fibrous tissue; *e*, superior retrodiscal lamina (elastic); *f*, inferior retrodiscal lamina (collagenous); *g*, retrodiscal loose connective tissue; *h*, posterior capsular ligament (collagenous); *i*, condylar axis of rotation; *j*, discal collateral ligament (collagenous); *k*, superior lateral pterygoid muscle; *l*, inferior lateral pterygoid muscle; *m*, anterior capsular ligament (collagenous); *x*, posterior margin of condylar articular facet. Note that the inclination of the articular eminence is about 52 degrees from the horizontal supra-articular crest.

so by exerting antagonistic elastic traction on the disc in a posterior direction.

The craniomandibular articulation, therefore, should be visualized as a bilateral sliding joint, supported by the temporomandibular ligaments and manipulated by the masticatory musculature. Each lateral portion is a compound joint with its articular disc serving as an active bone; the mandible is attached to the cranium by means of disc-condyle complexes that act like hinges. All functioning of the craniomandibular articulation involves an intricate mixture of sliding and hinge movement bilaterally. The articular discs play the dominant biomechanical role.

Interarticular Pressure

The interarticular pressure in the temporomandibular joint, as in other synovial joints, varies considerably during normal functioning of the mandible. The interarticular pressure remains relatively constant during empty-mouth movements—nonchewing, nonstressed, nonresistance movements. Interarticular pressure during such movement is the result of muscle tonus modified by the negative effect of gravity, due to myotatic reflex activity. Variation in interarticular pressure results from active contraction of masticatory muscles when the teeth meet resistance.

Biting against resistance during a power stroke induces torque forces in the mandible that are transmitted to the temporomandibular joints. *The pressure in the joint on the chewing side decreases, while the pressure in the joint on the opposite side increases* (Fig 3–2). This concept is consistent with electromyographic findings.[2] It is consistent with radiographically apparent changes in the width of the articular disc space during power strokes.[6] It is also consistent with clinical diagnostic observations that minor discal interference during translatory movement often may be reduced, or even eliminated, by biting against resistance on the symptomatic side. The reverse may be true of biting against resistance on the nonsymptomatic side.

Joint Stability

As with other synovial joints, stability of the articulating surfaces is maintained by sharp contact at all times—while at rest, during relaxed movements, and during power strokes.[7] Loss of contact constitutes disarticulation. The articular discs play the essential role in maintaining sharp contact of the articulating parts in the craniomandibular articulation.

NORMAL DISC FUNCTION DURING EMPTY-MOUTH MOVEMENTS

Most functioning of the craniomandibular articulation occurs with minimal muscular activity. Consequently, interarticular pressure remains constant bilaterally as muscle tonus provides continuous sharp contact of the articulating parts. Active contraction of the various muscles is limited to that required for mandibular movement in the absence of resistance and stress. Power strokes and maximum intercuspation do not enter the picture. Such functioning is referred to as *empty-mouth movements*.

The dentition has little, if any, influence on such movements under normal circumstances because the teeth are not occluded firmly. Any contact of the teeth is very light and does not tend to alter the positioning force of

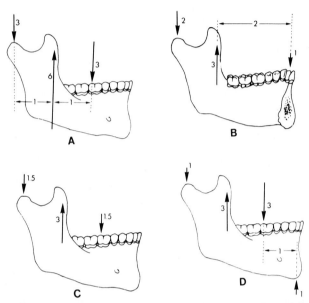

Fig 3–2.—Biomechanics of the mandible in the lateral projection. *A,* no distinction is made between forces on the ipsilateral and contralateral sides. The perpendicular distance between the resultant muscle force and the bite force is 1 unit. The perpendicular distance between the resultant muscle force and the condylar reaction force is also 1 unit. Six units of muscle force yield 3 units of both bite force and condylar force. *B,* forces acting on the contralateral side of the mandible. The muscle force on the contralateral side is divided into condylar reaction force and a force that is transmitted to the ipsilateral side through the mandibular symphysis. The distance between the contralateral resultant muscle force and the symphysis is 2 units. Three units of muscle force yield 2 units of condylar reaction force and 1 unit of force transmitted through the symphysis. *C,* forces acting on the ipsilateral side without consideration of the force being transmitted through the symphysis from the contralateral side. The 3 units of resultant muscle force are divided equally between the bite force and the condylar reaction force. *D,* forces acting on the ipsilateral side. The distance between the force acting through the symphysis and the bite force is 1 unit. The 3 units of muscle force on the ipsilateral side and the 1 unit of force acting through the symphysis yield 1 unit of reaction force and 3 units of bite force. (From Hylander W.L., in Sarnat B.G., Laskin D.M. (eds.): *The Temporomandibular Joint,* ed. 3, 1979. Courtesy of Charles C Thomas, Publisher, Springfield, Ill.)

muscle action. Even with swallowing, light occlusion of the teeth usually does not bring into play the overriding effect of firmly articulated inclined planes of teeth. Only empty-mouth clenching of the teeth (maximum intercuspation) initiates the determinant positioning force exerted by tooth form. Although occasional clenching of the teeth is normal, just as is occasional yawning, clenching in excess of that needed to maintain the resting length of the lateral pterygoid muscles constitutes bruxism. Its effect on the articular discs will be considered subsequently.

Since empty-mouth functioning involves neither power strokes nor maximum intercuspation, articular disc movement is needed chiefly to facilitate two biomechanical functions, namely, separation of the jaws and translation of the condyle. The continuing effect of muscle tonus furnishes adequate stability in the joint by maintaining sharp contact of the articulating parts.

Disc Action for Separation of Jaws

Separation of the chewing frames that support the teeth is accomplished by rotation of the condyles *in the articular discs.* The relative movement in the disc-condyle complex is that of rotation of the disc posteriorly on the condyle (Fig 3–3). The limit of such rotation is the posterior border of the condylar articular facet—a limit that seldom is reached in the absence of translation of the condyle. Pure rotatory opening does not occur frequently, unless volition is involved. It has been established that some degree of translation almost invariably occurs when the jaws are separated.[5]

Disc Action During Translatory Cycle

Nearly every movement of the mandible involves part of the translatory cycle in addition to separation of the jaws. Normal functioning is a combination of both factors. The translatory cycle movements within the joint are much the same whether due to opening, protrusion, or lateral excursion. Straight-line opening and straight-line protrusion produce nearly

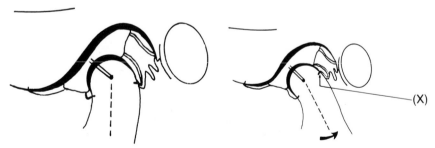

Fig 3–3.—Effect of separating the jaws on movement within the disc-condyle complex. *Left,* resting closed position of the joint. *Right,* rotation of the condyle in the articular disc to separate the jaws. Note that the relationship between disc and eminence does not change. Rotation of the condyle moves the posterior margin of the condylar articular facet *(x)* closer to the posterior edge of the articular disc. This amounts to posterior rotatory movement in the disc-condyle complex.

identical and bilaterally symmetric translatory cyclic movements in the joint. Deviated or deflected movements produce compensatory asymmetry of movement. Lateral excursion produces maximum asymmetry: the disc-condyle complex on the working side pivots, while that on the balancing side translates. The translating disc-condyle complex during lateral excursion moves slightly medially as it descends the articular eminence. This difference is not grossly significant except that it restrains somewhat the extent of anterior movement in the forward phase of the translatory cycle. This observation is readily apparent radiographically; the normal extent of forward movement of the condyle in lateral excursion is invariably *less* than in opening or protrusion (Fig 3–4).

SLIDING OF THE DISC.—As the forward phase of the cycle takes place, the upper surface of the articular disc slides down the articular eminence, rounds the crest, and moves forward along its anterior plane. During the return phase of the cycle, the upper surface of the disc retraces the sliding movement back to the resting or lightly occluded position.

If the upper articular facet were entirely flat, so that sliding between the disc-condyle complex and temporal bone were straight, the sliding movement between the two articulating surfaces would be a simple bodily movement: the disc and condyle would move in unison and in the same amount. This, however, is not the case. First, the articular eminence slopes downward, then it levels at the crest, followed by a slightly upward sloping of the anterior surface of the eminence. In order for the upper surface of the disc-condyle complex to maintain full surface contact with the temporal

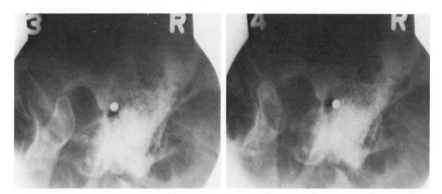

Fig 3–4.—Transparietal radiographs of temporomandibular joint in lateral position *(left)* and open position *(right)*. Note that in lateral position the condyle moves to the crest of the articular eminence. In open position it moves well beyond the crest, a considerably greater distance than in lateral position. This is a normal movement pattern.

articular facet, *the disc must rotate anteroposteriorly on the condyle.*

It will be seen, therefore, that in order to maintain surface contact of the articulating parts during the translatory cycle, the disc rotates posteriorly on the condyle as the disc-condyle complex moves forward in relationship to the articular eminence. This posterior rotation continues as the crest is reached and is greatest as the forward phase of the cycle is completed (Fig 3–5). This maneuver causes the bodily forward movement of the articular disc to be considerably less than that of the condyle. This observation has been erroneously interpreted as evidence of sliding movement between the condyle and disc—a condition rendered anatomically impossible by the discal collateral ligaments as long as they remain functional. During the return phase, the disc rotates anteriorly until the cycle is completed, thus returning the disc-condyle complex back to the resting or lightly occluded position. *It should be noted that the greater the inclination of the articular*

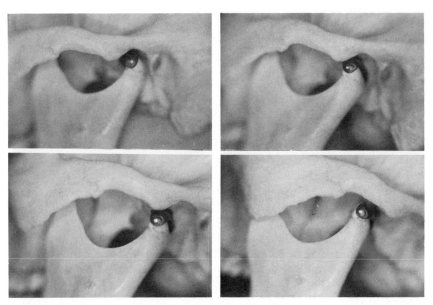

Fig 3–5.—Photographs of dry skull with a simulated articular disc hinged on condyle to illustrate posterior rotation of the articular disc on the condyle during forward translatory movement of the disc-condyle complex (opening movement). *Top left,* joint in resting closed position. *Top right,* condyle moved halfway toward crest of eminence. *Bottom left,* condyle at crest of articular eminence. *Bottom right,* condyle at full forward translatory position. Note that as condyle moves anteriorly, the articular disc rotates posteriorly on the condyle. Owing to this rotatory movement, during forward translation the articular disc moves a shorter distance than the condyle.

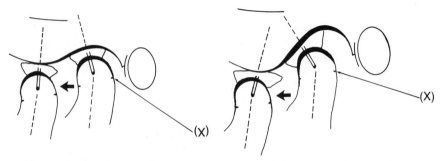

Fig 3–6.—Effect of inclination of articular eminence on amount of rotation of the articular disc during forward translatory movement. *Left,* inclination of articular eminence about 28 degrees from horizontal supra-articular crest. *Right,* inclination of articular eminence about 52 degrees from horizontal supra-articular crest. Note that as disc-condyle complex moves forward (as in a protrusive movement), the articular disc rotates posteriorly on the condyle. By comparing the movement of the posterior edge of the articular disc toward the posterior margin of the condylar articular facet *(x),* note that the amount of such rotation in the 28-degree joint is considerably less than in the 52-degree joint. The steeper the inclination of the articular eminence, the greater the rotatory movement in the disc-condyle complex during translatory movements.

eminence, *the greater the amount of posterior rotation of the articular disc on the condyle* (Fig 3–6).

An important key to the amount of rotation of the disc (in order to maintain continuous surface contact between the disc-condyle complex and the temporal articular facet during the translatory cycle) is the inclination and total height of the articular eminence. Because of the rotatory movement of the disc posteriorly on the condyle as the whole complex moves forward, the total bodily movement of the condyle in relationship to the temporal bone exceeds that of the articular disc. *This difference increases as the inclination and height of the articular eminence increases.*

The clinical significance of this information is that the greater the inclination and height of the articular eminence, the greater the demand for rotation of the disc to accomplish smooth, silent, unobstructed translatory movements. *Extreme inclination and height of the eminence predispose to disc interference problems, and once these problems come into existence, the effects of inclination and height are augmented.* Accurate knowledge of the inclination and height of the eminence, therefore, is important in evaluating function and dysfunction of the joints. The rotatory movement of the disc on the condyle to facilitate translatory movement must be understood and appreciated.

Combined Separation of Jaws and Condylar Translation

During protrusion and lateral excursion, when separation of the jaws is minimal, the total rotation of disc on condyle is only that required to maintain surface contact between the sliding parts. Normal opening of the mouth entails, in addition, a large component of rotation sufficient to achieve separation of the jaws. As already mentioned, rotation for both purposes is in the same posterior direction, relative to disc-condyle position. With wide opening, therefore, the limit of posterior rotation of the disc may be reached, this being determined by the posterior border of the condylar articular facet. Once this limit is reached, further rotation of the disc on the condyle is impossible. This constitutes the limit of *normal* opening. Overextended opening of the mouth can move the disc-condyle complex forward beyond this point, but such movement must take place without benefit of articular disc rotation that is essential to surface-to-sur-

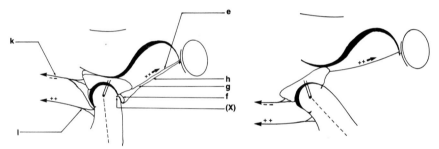

Fig 3–7.—Comparison of maximum normal forward translatory movement and subluxation of disc-condyle complex. *Left,* maximum normal forward translatory movement (*e,* superior retrodiscal lamina; *f,* inferior retrodiscal lamina; *g,* retrodiscal loose connective tissue; *h,* posterior capsular ligament; *k,* superior lateral pterygoid muscle; *l,* inferior lateral pterygoid muscle; *x,* posterior margin of condylar articular facet). Maximum normal forward translatory movement is reached when articular disc is rotated posteriorly until its edge reaches the posterior margin of the condylar articular facet *(x),* thus arresting further rotatory movement of the disc on the condyle. In this position the dominant traction force on the articular disc is in a posterior direction due to the fully stretched superior retrodiscal lamina *(e)* against the inactive relaxed superior lateral pterygoid muscle *(k).* The dominant traction force on the condyle is in an anterior direction, owing to the actively contracted inferior lateral pterygoid muscle *(l)* against the taut posterior capsular ligament *(h). Right,* subluxated disc-condyle complex. Opening beyond the maximum normal forward translatory movement causes the disc-condyle complex to rotate on itself because of the restraining effect of the posterior capsular ligament and arrested rotatory movement in the complex. As a result, the disc-condyle complex skids bodily along the articular eminence in a rough, noisy, jerking movement.

face contact of the articular parts. Since the disc cannot rotate farther, continued movement of the complex forward causes it to skid bodily along the upper articular surface (Fig 3–7).

Pivoting of Condyle

During a lateral excursion, the disc-condyle complex pivots on the working side, while translating on the balancing side. The pivoting (trochoid) movement takes place between the upper surface of the disc and the temporal articular facet. Initially, the vertical axis of rotation passes through the center of the condyle. But, as the lateral pole rotates posteriorly, it becomes restrained by the inner horizontal fibers of the temporomandibular ligament. This shifts the vertical axis of rotation outward to the lateral pole of the pivoting condyle.[1] Normally this trochoid movement meets no resistance or interference during empty-mouth movements because of the low interarticular pressure.

NORMAL DISC FUNCTION IN RESPONSE TO BITING STRESS

When the masticatory muscles force the mandible against resistance, as happens in prehension, incising, and grinding, the biomechanics of the temporomandibular joint change. The conditions that affect articular disc function are different from those that exist during empty-mouth movements. Human activities have imposed many nonmasticatory functions upon the jaws and teeth. However, the jaws and teeth appear to behave in much the same way, although the time element may be different. Holding a pipe between the teeth simulates biting against any hard object except that it is a prolonged activity.

Power Strokes

A complete power stroke differs from an empty-mouth translatory cycle in two ways: (1) at some point during the return phase of the cycle, resistance is met and continues to some extent for the remainder of the return phase, and (2) the cycle terminates in maximum intercuspation of the teeth instead of in the resting position or in light occlusal contact.

RESISTANCE DURING RETURN PHASE.—Effects of biting against resistance do not involve tooth form as such, but the added sensory input from stimulated periodontal receptors may modify guidance of muscle action in directing the chewing stroke to completion.

The particular point in the return phase at which the biomechanical factors change is determined by how far the jaws are separated when the object is engaged. This relates to the size of the object grasped and where it is located in the mouth. The continuance of such factors through the return phase of the translatory cycle depends on the intent of the effort (whether to hold, crack, bite through, incise, or grind) as well as the ability of the apparatus to accomplish such intent. The flexion or nociceptive reflex helps protect components of the system from injury: sudden, unexpected, painful encounters of the teeth cause immediate arrest of activity in the power muscles with simultaneous contraction of antagonists.

Several factors influence the degree of biomechanical change that occurs during a power stroke. These factors include the size and consistency of the object of resistance, the intent behind the stroke, the speed of the stroke, the distance between the object and the joint (the load moment), and the torquing effect of unilateral biting stress.

From radiographic evidence, it is known that biting hard against resistance causes perceptible widening of the articular disc space on the biting side. This widening continues in a diminishing way until the object is penetrated and the teeth come into full occlusion.[5] In order to prevent separation and, therefore, disarticulation of the parts, biomechanical requirements demand that continuing firm contact be maintained during this period of instability. As described by Sicher, sharp contact of the articulating surfaces results from contraction of the superior lateral pterygoid muscle which exerts both a strong holding action on the condylar neck to control the movement of the disc-condyle complex during the return phase of the power stroke, and *strong anterior traction on the articular disc itself,* thus firmly rotating a thicker portion of disc into the widened articular disc space (Fig 3–8). This particular muscular activity has been confirmed electromyographically.[3, 4]

During power strokes, therefore, the articular discs take on an essential, special function, that of rotating anteroposteriorly in order to maintain constant joint stability during fluctuations of interarticular pressure (by firmly filling the articular disc space at all times). *The actual position of the disc in relationship to the condylar facet at any particular time is determined by the width of the articular disc space,* which in turn reflects the interarticular pressure.

MAXIMUM INTERCUSPATION. — During empty-mouth movements, the interarticular pressure remains relatively constant, being that of muscle tonus primarily. Thus, the articular disc space remains uniform, and little anteroposterior rotation of the disc for this purpose is required. During power strokes, however, the decreased interarticular pressure on the biting side and increased pressure on the opposite side cause changes in the articular disc spaces that are compensated for by rotatory disc movements. Narrow-

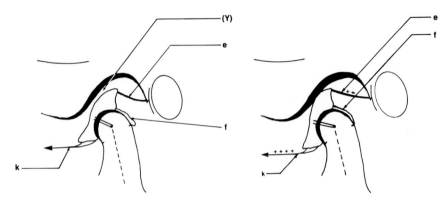

Fig 3-8.—Movements in the disc-condyle complex generated by a power stroke against resistance. *Left,* power stroke against resistance increases the width of the articular disc space on the biting side, as indicated at *y*. This occurs in response to negative interarticular pressure in the ipsilateral joint as the biting force is torqued through the mandibular symphysis to the contralateral joint. *Right,* a thicker portion of articular disc is rotated forward between the separated articular surfaces, thus maintaining firm surface contact between the articulating parts to adequately stabilize the joint during the remainder of the power stroke. This rotatory movement of the articular disc is accomplished by strong active contraction of the superior lateral pterygoid muscle *(k)*, thus overcoming the posterior traction of the stretched superior retrodiscal lamina *(e)*, which dominates the position of the disc during the forward phase of translation until a power stroke begins. Note that the amount of forward rotation of the articular disc is limited by the inferior retrodiscal lamina *(f)*, thus preventing functional dislocation.

ing of the space causes the articular disc to assume a more centered position, thus placing a thinner portion of disc between the condyle and articular eminence. This occurs in the joint on the side opposite to where the resistance is encountered and in both joints when the teeth are brought into maximum intercuspation. Following maximum intercuspation, the muscles relax, thus decreasing the interarticular pressure and proportionately increasing the width of the articular disc space. As the disc space widens slightly, the forward pull of the superior lateral pterygoid muscle (due to muscle tonus) rotates the disc anteriorly to bring a slightly thicker portion of disc firmly into the space.

When the teeth come into maximum intercuspation, the occlusion becomes a force that must be taken into account. If the condylar position dictated by the dentition is identical to that already imposed by muscle action, then only increased interarticular pressure is present, because no movement is involved. The joints ordinarily sustain such pressure very well, and no damage results. But, if the dentition-dictated position of the condyle varies from that imposed by muscle action, movement of the condyle takes place, and such movement is under increasing interarticular pressure. As the articular disc moves under pressure against the temporal articular facet, frictional abuse may predispose to damage. Once the disc becomes firmly anchored by the effect of friction, further movement forced by the dentition tends to displace the disc and condyle, thus placing considerable strain on the discal collateral ligaments. Movement under such conditions may cause injury, the severity of which depends on such factors as the force and extent of movement, the direction, frequency, and duration of such movement, and the structural form of the components involved.

Empty-Mouth Clenching

Bruxism is another situation in which stressed movement influences articular disc function. Normally, the teeth are brought into full occlusion only momentarily during chewing strokes or when the teeth are occasionally clenched. Even when some occlusal disharmony is present, the joints ordinarily are able to tolerate such demands of function without sustaining appreciable damage. But, if the teeth are clenched frequently or for long periods of time, various muscle effects and deleterious changes may result. If gross occlusal disharmony is present, the danger increases materially. The same may be said for habitual biting and chewing with excessive force.

Clinical Significance of Stressed Movements

The movements of the articular disc in response to varying interarticular pressure between the articulating parts of the joint should be understood and appreciated, for in them is a key to understanding masticatory function and dysfunction. Generally, such movements of the disc are too subtle to be noticed. In disc-interference disorders of the joint, however, their significance becomes important indeed.

COMPOSITE MANDIBULAR MOVEMENTS

When viewed grossly, as, for example, radiographically, it would *appear* that, with opening and closing the mouth, the condyle simply rotates to separate the jaws and slides forward on the temporal bone. With protrusion, the condyle *appears* to rotate only very slightly but slides boldly forward on the temporal bone. Lateral excursion *appears* to move similarly, except unilaterally. Such visualization of temporomandibular movements would be accurate, if the condyle articulated with the temporal bone with an interposed meniscus. This, however, is not the case—the articular disc is not a meniscus.

The gross movement of the osseous parts (as viewed radiographically) *constitutes only a portion of the intricate movements that take place in the temporomandibular joint during normal functioning.* Two distinct types of rotatory movement take place, namely, rotation of the *condyle in the articular disc* and rotation of the *disc on the condyle.* Separation of the jaws calls for rotation of the condyle in the disc. As this rotation takes place, the posterior border of the condylar articular facet comes closer to the posterior edge of the articular disc. In relationship to the disc-condyle complex, the articular disc rotates *posteriorly.* In order to maintain continuous surface contact of the sliding parts during translatory movement forward, the articular disc rotates on the condyle: the steeper and higher the eminence, the greater the amount of rotation. This rotation also brings the posterior border of the condylar articular facet closer to the posterior border of the disc. In relationship to the disc-condyle complex, the disc rotates *posteriorly.* The more the condyle is moved anteriorly, the greater the rotation of the disc on the condyle. The limit of normal translation of the condyle is reached when the posterior edge of the articular disc comes in contact with the posterior border of the condylar articular facet. Protrusion and lateral excursion require only minimal rotation of the condyle in the disc but maximal rotation of the disc on the condyle. Normal opening, however, requires much of both types of rotatory movement.

Another requirement for rotation of the articular disc on the condyle has to do with variation in interarticular pressure in response to masticatory stresses. As pressure decreases and the articular disc space widens, the articular disc is rotated forward to fill it with a thicker portion of disc and, thus, maintain sharp contact of the articulating parts. Conversely, when the interarticular pressure increases perceptibly and the articular disc space decreases in width, the articular disc rotates posteriorly, leaving a thinner portion of disc in the space. The limit of this particular movement is reached when the disc is completely centered with its thinnest portion interposed between the condyle and temporal bone. Such demands for rotation of the disc on the condyle occur during power strokes and on maximum intercuspation of the teeth.

STRUCTURAL LIMITATIONS ON ARTICULAR DISC FUNCTION

Movement between the articular disc and condyle is restricted to hinge action (rotation) in the sagittal plane by the shape of the articulating surfaces and the presence of collateral ligaments that attach the disc to the lateral poles of the condyle. The whole disc-condyle complex is free to move against the temporal bone in all directions, since the articulating surfaces are relatively flat and not inhibited by ligamentous restraints.

Posterior rotation of the disc on the condyle is limited by the range of the lower segment of the anterior capsular ligament. The maximum useful range of movement is reached when the posterior edge of the articular disc arrives at the posterior border of the condylar articular facet. Rotation is arrested when this limit is reached, thus constituting the limit of normal forward translatory movement of the disc-condyle complex. The higher and steeper the articular eminence, the more rotation of the disc is required, and the more likely it is this limitation will be reached.

Anterior rotation of the articular disc on the condyle is limited to that permitted by the inferior retrodiscal lamina. During normal functioning of the temporomandibular joint, this restriction is rarely reached. In case of dislocation, however, this structure restricts the extent of anterior rotatory prolapse of the disc on the condyle.

DETERMINANTS OF DISC-CONDYLE POSITION

In addition to the collateral ligaments that prevent sliding movement between the articular disc and the condyle, two *active forces* relative to disc-condyle position are present, namely, the anterior traction exerted by the superior lateral pterygoid muscle and the posterior traction exerted by the elasticity of the superior retrodiscal lamina. In the resting position, the muscular pull is dominant so that at rest, the disc is rotated anteriorly as far as the width of the articular disc space permits. In forward translation, however, the extended superior retrodiscal lamina becomes dominant, thus causing the articular disc to occupy the most posterior rotatory position on the condyle permitted by the width of the articular disc space. The superior lateral pterygoid muscle remains inactive during the forward phase of the translatory cycle, as well as during the critical shift from forward movement to the return phase. Thus, stability is ensured during this critical turn-around period by the maintenance of sharp contact between the articulating parts. Being firmly rotated posteriorly, the disc resists spontaneous anterior dislocation. If the superior lateral pterygoid muscle should contract prematurely at this critical time, the articular disc would be rotated anteriorly, and dislocation could result. *The primary function of the superior retrodiscal lamina is to resist spontaneous dislocation of the articular disc at the most forward point of the translatory cycle.*

During empty-mouth movements, when interarticular pressure remains nearly constant and the width of the articular disc space remains uniform, the effect of muscle tonus in the superior lateral pterygoid muscle continues to be greater than the effect exerted by the elasticity of the superior retrodiscal lamina. This keeps the articular disc in the most forward rotatory position permitted by the width of the articular disc space. During forward translation, this changes gradually as the superior retrodiscal lamina is stretched. At the full forward position, the lamina is dominant, thus rotating the disc posteriorly and preventing dislocation. This condition prevails until the disc-condyle complex has begun its return phase. Then, the shift in dominance of force gradually changes back to that of the muscle, thus ensuring that the disc occupy its most anterior position on the condyle permitted by the articular disc space. This delicate balance depends on precise muscular coordination. Its significance in normal functioning of the joint should be understood and appreciated. In this way, stability of the joint is maintained during the complete translatory cycle by continuous sharp contact of the articulating parts.

During a power stroke, which *begins well after the extreme forward point of translation has been reached and the disc-condyle complex is safely on its return phase,* a marked change in interarticular pressure occurs, which in turn alters the width of the disc space. On the biting side, the disc space widens perceptibly. If no new force entered the picture at this moment, the posterior traction exerted by the stretched superior retrodiscal lamina would tend to dislocate the articular disc posteriorly (if the disc space widened sufficiently). But, as the elevator muscles contract to execute the power stroke, contraction of the superior lateral pterygoid muscle takes place and exerts strong holding action on the mandibular condyle. The separate attachment of this muscle to the articular disc immediately overcomes the effect of the stretched superior retrodiscal lamina and rotates the articular disc anteriorly, thus bringing it firmly into the widened articular disc space. In this way stability of the joint is maintained by sharp contact of the articulating surfaces.

The contraction of the superior lateral pterygoid muscle continues throughout the remainder of the power stroke. It is especially active when the teeth are firmly brought into maximum intercuspation. At this time, interarticular pressure is greatest and the articular disc space is thinnest. The articular disc is centered on the condyle, with the thinnest portion interposed between the condyle and articular eminence. With the disc thus firmly wedged between the osseous surfaces and the superior lateral pterygoid muscle strongly contracted, *joint stability is maximal just as occlusion of the teeth takes place*. Then, as the elevator and superior lateral pterygoid muscles relax and the mandible assumes a position of rest, a state of muscular equilibrium represented by muscle tonus prevails.

With the normal relaxation of the elevator and lateral pterygoid muscles following maximum intercuspation, the resting condition of the joint is reestablished. With decrease in interarticular pressure, slight widening of the articular disc space takes place. The superior lateral pterygoid muscle rotates the articular disc anteriorly to fill the slightly widened disc space, as muscle tonus exceeds the traction of the relaxed nonstretched superior retrodiscal lamina. As this occurs, synovial fluid is brought in between the articulating surfaces and the joint is lubricated and made ready for the next movement.

Even in the presence of anteroposterior traction forces exerted on the articular disc, the determinant of position between disc and condyle at any given time is the *width of the disc space*, as determined by joint pressure. The anterior and posterior traction forces on the disc are needed only to maintain continued sharp contact of the articulating parts under all conditions of joint use. Knowledge of the functioning of the articular disc is necessary for correct clinical evaluation of the various conditions of articular disc interference that constitute many temporomandibular disorders.

REQUIREMENTS FOR NORMAL DISC FUNCTIONING

In order for articular disc movements to remain free from interference, several conditions should prevail:

1. The articular surfaces should be smooth, rounded, structurally compatible in shape, and adequately lubricated.

2. Movements of the right and left joints should be reasonably symmetric.

3. Sliding movement between articulating surfaces should not take place when interarticular pressure is sufficient to cause friction.

4. Except in very flat joints, no appreciable movement between the unclenched and clenched occluded-joint positions should occur as maximum intercuspation takes place.

5. Precise coordination of muscle action should prevail at all times.

6. Joint function should be habitually restrained within the structural capability of the joints.

When such conditions do not prevail, discal interference may result. This can induce acute muscle disorders or cause damage to components of the joint.

CONDITIONS THAT MAY CAUSE DISC INTERFERENCE

Some of the causes of articular disc interference are:

1. Very steeply inclined articular eminences.

2. Excessive speed, force, or extent of jaw movement.

3. Excessive passive interarticular pressure.

4. Arrested or otherwise abnormal movement in the opposite joint.

5. Structural incompatibility between the articulating surfaces of the joint or between the right and left joints.

6. Chronic occlusal disharmony that causes gross movement between the unclenched and clenched occluded positions of the joint.

7. Damaged temporal articular facet at the closed position of the joint.

8. Damaged temporal articular facet along the articular eminence.

9. Damaged disc-condyle complex: *(a)* adhesions between the articular disc and condyle, *(b)* damaged articular disc, *(c)* damaged discal collateral ligaments, *(d)* damaged superior retrodiscal lamina.

REFERENCES

1. Du Brul E.L.: *Sicher's Oral Anatomy*, ed. 7. St. Louis, C.V. Mosby Co., 1980.
2. Hylander W.L.: Functional anatomy, in Sarnat B.G., Laskin D.M. (eds.): *The Temporomandibular Joint*, ed. 3. Springfield, Ill., Charles C Thomas, Publisher, 1979, pp. 85–113.
3. Lipke D.P., Gay T., Gross B.D., et al.: An electromyographic study of the human lateral pterygoid muscle. *J. Dent. Res.* 56B:230, 1977.
4. McNamara J.A. Jr.: The independent functions of the two heads of the lateral pterygoid muscle. *Am. J. Anat.* 138:197, 1973.
5. Nevakari K.: An analysis of the mandibular movement from rest to occlusal position. *Acta Odont. Scan.*, vol. 14, suppl. 19, 1956.
6. Scully J.J.: *Cinefluorographic Studies of the Masticatory Movements of the Human Mandible*. Thesis, University of Illinois, 1959.
7. Sicher H.: Functional anatomy of the temporomandibular joint, in Sarnat B.G. (ed.): *The Temporomandibular Joint*, ed. 2. Springfield, Ill., Charles C Thomas, Publisher, 1964, pp. 28–58.

4 / Masticatory Muscle Function

MUSCLE ACTION is the source of power for all musculoskeletal functioning. Stability, position, and movement are determined by the skeletal musculature, which is coordinated by efferent neural impulses from the CNS. Incoming information is supplied by a continuous inflow of monitoring afferent neural impulses from muscles and other peripheral structures. To understand masticatory function requires some knowledge of muscle structure and behavior.

Muscles do not act singly. Useful muscle action is concerted and purposeful. Agonist muscles cooperate to perform an action; antagonist muscles act in opposition to agonist muscles and produce the control and graduated action necessary for useful movements. No specific function can be assigned to a single muscle without due consideration for the cooperative and opposing actions of other muscles.

STRUCTURE

Skeletal muscles are composed of many bundles (fasciculi) of fibers, each bundle containing a number of parallel fibers. A muscle fiber consists of sarcoplasm, which is composed of alternate light and dark portions that account for its striated appearance. Each fiber is made up of myofibrils that presumably represent the contractile elements of the muscle. Each fiber is surrounded by a delicate elastic sheath, called sarcolemma, which gives muscle tissue some elasticity.

The basic unit of the neuromuscular system is the *motor unit,* which consists of muscle fibers and a single motor neuron. The number of fibers contained within a motor unit is variable and seems to relate to the complexity of the motor action involved: the more precise the movement, the fewer fibers per motor neuron.

MUSCLE CONTRACTION

When stimulated by activity in the motor neuron, the fibers of a motor unit contract. When the stimulation ceases, the fibers relax. This operates on an all-or-none principle. Contractile activity results from active groups of muscle fibers intermingled with inactive groups throughout the muscle. The activity shifts from group to group so that alternating periods of activity

55

and rest preclude the fatiguing of any particular group. The degree of contractile activity of a muscle depends on the relative number of muscle fibers active at a given time. Muscle fatigue results when the demand for contractile activity exceeds the capability of group interchange within the muscle.

Contractile activity may shorten the muscle under constant loading, thus inducing skeletal movement. Such contraction is termed *isotonic*. Contractile activity may increase tension within the muscle while maintaining a constant muscle length, thus producing a holding action. Such contraction is termed *isometric*. Both types of contractile activity may occur in the same muscle, giving it great versatility. Coordinated muscle action consists of various combinations of such contractile activity in agonist and antagonist muscle groups.

Contractile activity may occur reflexly in automatic response to stimulation of receptors within the muscle and its tendinous attachments. Such reflex activity is somewhat self-regulatory and subject to the influence of other sensory input and to stimulation from the CNS. Contractile activity may follow preconditioned habit patterns, some of which may be so deeply ingrained as to induce nearly automatic and unconscious behavior. Contractile activity may occur in response to volition, which usually is capable of overriding habitual muscular activity.

Muscle Tonus

Muscle tonus may be defined as the resistance of the muscle to elongation or stretch. *Hypertonicity* refers to a relative increase in passive resistance to stretching the muscle; *hypotonicity* refers to a decreased passive resistance to stretch. Muscle tonus is based primarily on the myotatic or stretch reflex, as far as active contraction of muscle fibers is concerned. The sum total of muscle tonus includes the effect of the elastic properties of muscle tissue itself.

Muscle tonus is somewhat self-regulatory, through the positive action of elongated muscle spindles that reflexly cause the muscle to contract. This relieves the tension on those spindles. It is subject to the adjusting effect of fusimotor activity, which increases spindle sensitivity to stretch by its shortening effect on the spindles. Muscle tonus is influenced by afferent input from other sensory receptors, such as those of the skin and mucosa, as well as by action of the CNS relative to systemic factors, both psychic and somatic. Such extraneous influence may be excitatory or inhibitory.

Muscle tonus serves two purposes: (1) it furnishes the muscular activity needed to maintain sharp contact of the articulating parts in joints when at rest or under negative interarticular pressure imposed by the effect of gravity, and (2) it maintains the muscles in an optimum state of readiness for contraction.

Muscle Splinting

When a muscle or other component of the musculoskeletal system is injured or threatened, as perceived by proprioceptive and sensory input from those and adjacent structures, protective muscle splinting may occur. This consists of increased tonicity of the musculature that has to do with movement of the threatened part, as if to stabilize it in space. Hypertonicity induces discomfort when the involved muscles are actively contracted, the resulting pain acting as an effective deterrent or inhibitory influence on such contractile efforts. This effect frequently is accompanied by a sensation of muscular weakness (pseudoparalysis), which reinforces the inhibitory influence on movement of the injured part. But no structual muscular dysfunction occurs.

Muscle splinting is considered to be a protective mechanism within the physiologic range of normal skeletal muscle behavior. It is induced involuntarily and thought to be a response to altered environmental sensory and proprioceptive input. It is influenced by reaction of the higher centers to painful stimuli and feelings of change, danger, or threat. The condition usually returns to normal as soon as the injury or threat disappears. Protracted muscle splinting may terminate in muscle spasm.

Muscle Spasm

Muscle spasm is a sudden involuntary contraction of a muscle or group of muscles that are functionally related. It is attended by pain and interference with function, and it is manifested by involuntary rigidity, distortion, or movement. Clonic muscle spasm is of momentary duration; tonic spasm persists for a period of time. Cycling muscle spasm is protracted tonic spastic activity that becomes self-perpetuating, presumably as the result of pain incidental to continued spastic contraction of the muscle. Isometric spasm causes muscular rigidity with marked resistance to stretch; isotonic spasm causes shortening of the muscle, which produces distortion or skeletal movement.

Clinical Significance

On a clinical level, masticatory muscle contractions may be divided into involuntary responses and working movements. Involuntary responses include (1) *muscle tonus,* which is the continued but variable degree of contraction of resting muscles that furnishes stability to the craniomandibular articulation as well as a position of physiologic rest for the mandible, (2) *muscle splinting,* which is a temporary state of hypertonicity induced as a protective mechanism to stabilize the threatened part in space and deter movement by pain inhibition and a feeling of weakness, but which does not otherwise introduce any structural muscular dysfunction, and (3) *cycling muscle spasm,* which is a protracted self-perpetuating state of involuntary tonic contraction attended by pain with all use and structural muscular dysfunction and which is expressed in rigidity or shortening of the muscle in spasm. It should be noted that these clinical effects differ largely in the degree of involuntary contraction of the muscles and, therefore, may not be differentiated with precision.[1] But, since treatment differs considerably, they should be identified *if possible.* Working movements include (1) voluntary conscious mandibular movements and (2) semiautomatic habitual chewing movements based on central patterns and guided by proprioceptive and sensory afferent input.

INNERVATION OF MUSCLES

Neural pathways subserving the masticatory musculature have to do with motor function. Each of the masticatory muscles receives branches from the mandibular division of the trigeminal nerve. The masseter is innervated by the masseteric nerve, the temporalis by three temporal nerves, the medial pterygoid by the medial pterygoid nerve, the lateral pterygoid muscle by the lateral pterygoid nerve, the mylohyoid by the mylohyoid nerve, and the anterior belly of the digastric muscle by a branch from the mylohyoid nerve. It should be noted that sensory pathways are not described.

Several considerations relative to the sensory innervation of the musculature should be kept in mind. It has been known for a long time that noxious stimulation of spinal ventral roots causes pain felt diffusely in the muscles innervated by those fibers.[2] It has recently been established that about 27% of the nerve fiber population contained within the spinal ventral (motor) roots consists of very fine nonmyelinated nerves, the function of which is not known but is very likely to conduct afferent impulses to the CNS.[3] It is known that at least some sensory fibers are contained within the motor nerves, since some sensory innervation to the temporomandibular capsule is by way of the masseteric and temporal (motor) nerves.[11] It also is known that the nerve cell bodies of proprioceptive fibers of the trigeminal nerve are not located with those of other sensory fibers in the dorsal root (gasserian) ganglion but rather are found in the mesencephalic nucleus located in the midbrain.[10] This would indicate that the afferent fibers relaying trigeminal proprioception need not pass through the dorsal sensory root. It is known that these[8] and other sensory fibers[5] are contained within the motor root. Taken together, this evidence justifies the assumption that sensory innervation to the masticatory muscles is by way of motor nerves to those muscles and that at least some of that sensory input is conducted to the CNS by way of the trigeminal motor, rather than sensory, root. Thus, some sensibility of the masticatory musculature may remain even though the trigeminal dorsal root is interrupted.

REFLEX ACTIVITY

Muscular activity is influenced by several known reflex mechanisms, namely, the myotatic, the nociceptive, and the inverse stretch reflexes.

Myotatic (Stretch) Reflex

When a muscle is stretched, it automatically contracts. The receptors for this reflex mechanism are the *muscle spindles*, which are mechanoreceptors arranged in parallel with the muscle fibers. They respond to *passive stretch* of the muscle. They cease to discharge if the muscle contracts isotonically, the spindles signaling muscle length. The neural relay is a monosynaptic circuit composed of two neurons, an afferent arm synapsing directly with a motoneuron that connects back to motor endplates of the muscle where the spindles are located. There is a reciprocal neural circuitry by which other muscles are simultaneously affected, namely, stimulation of agonist muscles and inhibitory influence on antagonist muscles. The muscle spindles are sensitive not only to structural length of muscle fibers but also to the rate of change of elongation as well. The sensitivity of the spindles to change is regulated by a biasing mechanism that establishes control over the effectiveness of myotatic reflex activity. Thus, one function of the muscle spindles is unconscious automatic control of muscular contractions during working movements and holding actions, according to the demands of function. They also serve to maintain stability of the parts at rest as an antigravity mechanism.

The myotatic reflex automatically operates when muscle stretch elongates the muscle spindles. This effect maintains sufficient muscle tonus to ensure continuous surface contact in synovial joints when the negative effect of gravity tends to separate them. With masticatory muscles, it is by the myotatic reflex that the weight of the mandible is overcome when the jaw is at rest. The stretching of elevator muscles due to mandibular weight would tend to separate the articulating parts of the temporomandibular joints. As the relaxed muscles stretch, the muscle spindles are elongated. As a result, the muscles contract until the tension of the spindles is equalized. The resulting increased tonicity in the elevator muscles maintains sharp contact of the articulating parts in the joints.

The myotatic reflex also influences muscle behavior during functional activities. This mechanism no doubt accounts for the *jaw-jerk reflex,* in which contraction of elevator muscles may be activated by downward tapping on the chin or the mandibular incisors or by tapping the point of insertion of the masseter muscle. It appears that such reflex activity may be influenced by associated sensory input from cutaneous, mucosal, and periodontal receptors.

It is important to know that myotatic reflex activity is absent in the lateral pterygoid and anterior digastric muscles. Presumably this is due to the dearth of spindles in those muscles. It should be obvious that such activity would disrupt masticatory movements. Such activity would be greatest when the lateral pterygoid muscles are stretched in the act of achieving maximum intercuspation of the teeth—a critical moment in the chewing stroke when smooth holding action of those muscles is of paramount importance. Reflex contraction of the muscle at that time would create conflictory forces completely disruptive to full occlusion of the teeth.

Nociceptive (Flexor, Flexion, Withdrawal) Reflex

When sudden, unexpected, *painful* stimulation of a part occurs, the muscles automatically react to cause withdrawal from the source of noxious input. This is called the nociceptive reflex. It is considered to be a protective mechanism to minimize injury. As related to the masticatory musculature, it accounts for the *jaw-opening reflex.* This is seen especially when one bites oneself or unexpectedly bites down hard on a rock; the jaws literally fly apart.

This reflex activity involves groups of muscles and is polysynaptic, the relay involving interneurons. In the jaw-opening reflex, active contraction of depressor and protractor muscles takes place with simultaneous relaxation of antagonist elevator muscles.

Since the nociceptive reflex is activated by painful stimulation, the receptor organs that initiate it no doubt are pain receptors. To what extent the receptors of the periodontal ligaments and the proprioceptors of the musculature and joints are involved is largely conjectural.

Inverse Stretch Reflex

When a muscle is stretched its full resting length, contraction ceases and the muscle relaxes fully. This response to *strong stretch* is known as the inverse stretch reflex. The receptors that initiate this activity are thought to be Golgi tendon organs, mechanoreceptors found in tendons of skeletal muscles arranged in series with the muscles. They are sensitive to mechanical distortion. Thus, they signal muscle tension and have inhibitory influence on muscle contraction.

The Golgi tendon organs likely play an important role in muscular activity as an inhibitory influence that helps to regulate contractile efforts of all types. Their activity influences, and is influenced by, the myotatic reflex mechanism. They no doubt have a role in coordinated muscle activity, as they are dominated not only by proprioceptive and sensory feedback mechanisms but by habitual and voluntary muscle action as well. Their protective effect to prevent injury as a result of hard muscular contraction is recognized. *The importance of this reflex in maintaining normal resting length of skeletal muscles should be understood.*

CONTRACTURE OF ELEVATOR MUSCLES.—The inverse stretch reflex causes a muscle to relax when it is elongated or stretched to its full length. If this normal physiologic maneuver is not permitted to take place occasionally, the muscle gradually shortens as its resting length decreases. The resulting contracture is called *myostatic contracture*.

An occasional yawn activates such a mechanism in the elevator muscles and is needed to prevent their contracture, which would reduce mouth-opening capability. If some condition is imposed on the elevator muscles that prevents normal action of the inverse stretch reflex, the extent to which the mouth can be opened is jeopardized. This can occur as the result of such structural conditions as intraoral adhesions, periarticular restraints to opening, intracapsular adhesions, or other arthropathy that restricts mouth opening. It may result from the inhibitory effects of protracted pain, habitual voluntary restraint of opening, or unduly protracted intermaxillary fixation.

ANTERIOR DRIFT OF EDENTULOUS MANDIBLE.—Another instance of inverse stretch reflex has to do with the lateral pterygoid muscles. An inverse stretch mechanism in those muscles is stimulated when they are fully stretched. This occurs with maximum intercuspation of the teeth. Just as an occasional yawn is necessary to maintain the full resting length of elevator muscles and, therefore, prevent loss of ability to open the mouth normally, so also is an occasional clenching of the teeth necessary to maintain full resting length of the lateral pterygoid muscles. This ensures the physiologic rest position of the mandible. Clenching the teeth occasionally is not only a normal physiologic activity of the masticatory muscles, it is a necessary one.

It should be noted that the effectiveness of activating the inverse stretch reflex to maintain the resting length of the lateral pterygoid muscles depends on the presence of teeth that can be fully occluded. Edentulousness eliminates the stretching of these muscles and the reflex mechanism cannot be activated in this condition. An artificial denture does not necessarily reestablish the reflex mechanism because the stretching force may be dissipated by the resilience of the supporting soft tissues or by actual movement of the denture on its supporting base. This is particularly true when the alveolar ridges are atrophic. Thus, edentulousness with or without artificial dentures may predispose to myostatic contracture of the lateral pterygoid muscles. Clinically this is recognized as a gradual progressive anterior drift of the mandible.

Swallowing (Palatal, Palatine) Reflex

Swallowing reflexly occurs when the palate is stimulated. This is known as the palatal or palatine reflex and occurs periodically under empty-mouth conditions as well as with eating. It may be induced voluntarily. This reflex is accompanied by closing the mouth, the so-called *jaw-closing reflex*, which can be induced independently by lightly stroking the tongue. These reflex activities appear to depend on superficial sensory receptors more than on muscle proprioceptors.

Gag (Pharyngeal) Reflex

Light touch or mild stimulation of the back of the pharynx may initiate more or less convulsive contraction of the constrictor muscle of the pharynx. This is known as the pharyngeal reflex. It may also be induced by light stimulation of the palate, tongue, and other soft tissues in the posterior part of the mouth. Psychic stimuli may initiate the reflex, as well. These reflex activities appear to depend largely on sensory receptors. The masticatory musculature participates considerably in this reflex activity.

EFFECT OF MASTICATORY MUSCLES ON MANDIBULAR MOVEMENT

Many years ago, anatomists, by employing principles of biomechanics, were able to discern the necessary actions of the various muscles that execute chewing movements. It is significant that all muscles that enter actively into mandibular functioning are innervated by the trigeminal nerve, the proprioceptors of which have their nerve cell bodies located in the mesencephalic nucleus of the midbrain, rather than in the gasserian ganglion, where the nerve cell bodies of other trigeminal sensory afferents are located.

Gross Mandibular Movements

Depressor action to open the mouth is executed by the mylohyoid and anterior digastric muscles. Elevator action to close the mouth is accomplished by the masseter, medial pterygoid, and temporalis muscles. Protrusive movement is performed by the inferior lateral pterygoid muscles, while retrusion is effected by contraction of portions of the temporalis and masseter muscles in conjunction with the anterior digastric muscles. The actual movements of opening, closing, protrusion, and lateral excursion, however, are considerably more complex than this. Both agonists and antagonists are involved to varying degrees. Power strokes for chewing differ from empty-mouth movements. Although the principles of biomechanics have afforded considerable insight into the action of various muscles during mandibular movements, it remained for electromyographic studies to confirm and refine understanding in this respect.

Translatory Cycle Movements

As summarized by Hylander,[6] electromyographic studies have contributed much to the knowledge of masticatory muscle action during chewing strokes. It has become evident that the masseter and medial pterygoid muscles serve primarily as sources of power, while the temporalis and lateral pterygoid muscles are important for stability and control. At rest and during empty-mouth translatory cycles, sharp contact of the articulating parts of the temporomandibular joints is maintained by the posterior fibers of the temporalis muscles, which exert vertical traction on the condyles to press them firmly against the posterior slope of the articular eminences. As the mouth opens and the condyles slide forward, these fibers swing forward to an oblique angle, thus holding the condyles up against the slope of the eminences. As this effect diminishes, contraction of the inferior lateral pterygoid muscles continues to maintain sharp stabilizing contact of the articulating parts during the forward phase of the translatory cycle.[4]

Electromyographic studies have shown that during the forward phase of a translatory cycle for opening the mouth, activity occurs first in the mylohyoids and then the digastrics, as the mandible is moved inferiorly. Next, activity occurs in the inferior lateral pterygoid muscles, as the condyles are moved anteriorly. *The superior lateral pterygoid muscles remain inactive throughout the forward phase of the cycle and do not show appreciable activity unless a power stroke is exercised.* If the translatory cycle is for a unilateral chewing stroke (lateral excursion), the activity in the inferior lateral pterygoid muscle on the chewing side slightly precedes that of the opposite side, presumably to reinforce its vital function of maintaining adequate stability in the chewing joint preparatory to the power stroke that is to follow. Then activity occurs in the inferior lateral pterygoid on the balancing side to move that condyle forward to accomplish a unilateral translatory cyclic movement.

In the absence of a power stroke, the return phase of the translatory cycle is initiated by activity in the medial pterygoid muscles, followed by the masseters. There is little increased activity in the temporalis and lateral pterygoid muscles, which continue their function of maintaining joint stability.

If resistance is met during the return phase and a power stroke ensues, marked activity occurs in the medial pterygoid and masseter muscles as they execute strong elevator force on the mandible. This is accompanied by marked activity in the *superior* lateral pterygoid muscles as a holding action on the mandibular condyles. They simultaneously provide strong anterior traction on the articular discs. If the power stroke is for bilateral incising of a food object held in the hand and assisted by the hand pulling anteriorly on the object, considerable activity of the posterior and middle temporalis fibers in conjunction with medial pterygoid and masseter activity takes place, presumably to counter the extrinsic anterior pulling force on the mandible exerted by the hand. If the power stroke is for unilateral chewing, the return phase of the translatory cycle is initiated by activity in the medial pterygoid muscles while the mandible still is being moved ipsilaterally. Next, activity increases in the temporalis on the chewing side, presumably to reinforce stability preparatory to the power stroke to follow. Then, activity is increased in the elevator muscles bilaterally, with only minor activity in the lateral pterygoids. As the power stroke begins, marked activity occurs in the temporalis on the chewing side, followed immediately by maximum activity in the other elevator muscles bilaterally. This is accompanied by marked activity in the superior lateral pterygoid muscles, the activity being greater on the chewing side.

Clinical Significance

Most of the information gained from electromyographic studies only confirms what had previously been discerned as the necessary functioning of the masticatory muscles. It graphically indicates the marked difference between power strokes and empty-mouth movements. It shows the effect of prehensile incising and of unilateral chewing movements. The most significant information has to do with lateral pterygoid muscle action. It points up the marked difference between the two heads of that muscle, which function almost as if they were completely separate muscles.[7, 9] The inferior heads, in conjunction with posterior temporalis fibers, furnish continuing stability to the joint. The inferior head protrudes the mandible and has much to do with executing the forward phase of the translatory cycle. Except during the full forward phase of the translatory cycle, the superior head furnishes anterior traction on the articular disc. This is accomplished by muscle tonus only, for this head shows no increased activity during the anterior movement of the condyle. The superior lateral pterygoid muscle, therefore, is not a protruder muscle. It does not draw the disc forward along with the condyle during translatory movement. Rather, it functions in such a way as to permit quite separate action of the articular disc and condyle. It becomes active only during power strokes.

Being attached to the condyle and articular disc separately, the superior lateral pterygoid muscle serves two functions: (1) it exerts strong holding action on the mandibular condyle, thus exercising control over the return movement of the disc-condyle complex during the power stroke, and (2) it exerts strong anterior traction on the articular disc, thus rotating it forward as far as the width of the disc space permits. This action takes place during the critical period when the width of the disc space is altered by the forces of the power stroke. In this way, the superior lateral pterygoid muscle furnishes stability to the joint during the power stroke, and this effect continues until maximum intercuspation is accomplished. Then, the elevator and lateral pterygoid muscles relax as the resting position of the mandible is assumed.

When the teeth are fully occluded, either at the completion of a power stroke or with empty-mouth clenching, strong positive anterior rotatory traction on the articular disc is present. This effect occurs in conjunction with strong elevator muscle action that holds the condyles firmly against the articular eminences. At this time, the interarticular pressure is greatest and the width of the articular disc spaces minimal. In this attitude, the articular discs are centered on the condyles, with the thinnest portion interposed between condyle and articular eminence.

Following maximum intercuspation, the superior lateral pterygoid and elevator muscles relax. As the interarticular pressure decreases, the articular disc space widens slightly. The traction force on the disc returns to that of muscle tonus in the superior lateral pterygoid muscle as opposed by the relaxed (nonstretched) superior retrodiscal lamina. Thus, the predominant muscle effect rotates the articular disc anteriorly as far as the width of the disc space permits.

It should be appreciated that this precisely coordinated action, which takes place every time the teeth are firmly occluded, can be severely interfered with by such factors as incoordinated muscle action, spasticity of muscles that interferes with normal activity, occlusal disharmony that sets up conflictory forces, and edentulousness. Interference with this mechanism may result in reactive muscle contractions of various types, strain and injury to resisting discal attachments, damage to the articular disc proper, and damage to the articular surfaces.

EFFECT OF MUSCLE ACTION ON ARTICULAR DISCS

Muscle action influences articular disc movements. During gross mandibular movements, rotation of the condyles in the discs (to separate the jaws) and rotation of the discs on the condyles (to maintain surface-to-surface contact between the discs and articular eminences during translatory movements) result from muscle action. It is also by muscle action that the articular disc spaces are kept filled properly as the width changes owing to fluctuation in interarticular pressure.

The superior lateral pterygoid muscle attaches to the articular disc. Owing to the effect of muscle tonus, it exerts sufficient rotatory force to keep the disc in the most anterior position permitted by the width of the articular disc space. This force is opposed by the superior retrodiscal lamina, the effect of which does not exceed that of muscle tonus except when it is extended during the full forward phase of a translatory cycle. Then, the posterior traction force of the retrodiscal tissue becomes dominant and rotates the disc posteriorly. In this way, the disc is protected against spontaneous anterior dislocation at the critical time when the translatory cycle shifts to the return phase.

During power strokes, change in the width of the articular disc space occurs as a result of altered interarticular pressure. As the elevator muscles contract to execute the biting stroke, simultaneous contraction of the superior lateral pterygoid muscle takes place. This rotates the disc anteriorly and firmly fills the disc space, thus maintaining joint stability. This effect continues throughout the power stroke and maximum intercuspation.

The effect of muscle action on articular disc function may be summarized as follows:

1. It maintains constant traction on the articular discs during empty-mouth movements, thus ensuring joint stability by keeping the articular discs rotated in the most forward position permitted by the width of the articular disc space at all times *except during the full forward phase of the translatory cycle*.

2. It provides strong positive anterior traction on the articular discs during power strokes and maximum intercuspation, thus maintaining joint stability when the disc spaces are altered in width by changing interarticular pressure.

REFERENCES

1. Bell W.E.: *Orofacial Pains, Differential Diagnosis*, ed. 2. Chicago, Year Book Medical Publishers, 1979.
2. Cailliet R.: *Neck and Arm Pain*. Philadelphia, F.A. Davis Co., 1964, p. 46.
3. Coggeshall R.E., Applebaum M.L., Fazen M., et al.: Unmyelinated axons in human ventral roots, a possible explanation for the failure of dorsal rhizotomy to relieve pain. *Brain* 98:157, 1975.
4. Du Brul E.L.: Origin and adaptations of the hominid jaw joint, in Sarnat B.G., Laskin D.M. (eds.): *The Temporomandibular Joint*, ed. 3. Springfield, Ill., Charles C Thomas, Publisher, 1979, pp. 5–34.
5. Hosobuchi Y.: The majority of unmyelinated afferent axons in human ventral roots probably conduct pain. *Pain* 8:167, 1980.
6. Hylander W.L.: Functional anatomy, in Sarnat B.G., Laskin D.M. (eds.): *The Temporomandibular Joint*, ed. 3. Springfield, Ill., Charles C Thomas, Publisher, 1979, pp. 85–113.
7. Lipke D.P., Gay T., Gross B.D., et al.: An electromyographic study of the human lateral pterygoid muscle. *J. Dent. Res.* 56B:230, 1977.
8. McIntyre A.K.: Afferent limb of the myotatic reflex arc. *Nature* 168:168, 1951.
9. McNamara J.A. Jr.: The independent functions of the two heads of the lateral pterygoid muscle. *Am. J. Anat.* 138:197, 1973.
10. Sicher H.: *Oral Anatomy*, ed. 3. St. Louis, C.V. Mosby Co., 1960, p. 356.
11. Thilander B.: Innervation of the temporomandibular joint capsule in man. *Trans. R. School Dent.* 7:1, 1961.

5 / Standards of Normal

EFFECTIVE MANAGEMENT of a temporomandibular complaint rests on knowledge of the individual patient's masticatory system. It matters little how the average craniomandibular articulation functions or what constitutes departure from normal for temporomandibular joints in general. Standards of normal should be derived and applied on an individual basis.

In order to establish a basis for judgment, it is important that we understand the functioning of the masticatory system in a way that allows for individual variations from average. Too rigid a concept of what constitutes normal should be avoided. Standards that are ideal should give way to standards that reflect considerable latitude in normal functioning of the masticatory system. Concepts of anatomical relationships without concern for their functional compatibility are neither useful nor practical.

CONCEPT OF DISC-CONDYLE COMPLEX FUNCTIONING

The key to the behavior of the craniomandibular articulation is the need for continuing surface contact of condyle, disc, and articular eminence under all conditions of normal functioning. Sliding movement that takes place between disc-condyle complex and articular eminence in any direction is functionally normal as long as it does not occur under pressure sufficient to cause frictional abuse to the moving surfaces. But sliding movement within the disc-condyle complex proper (i.e., between condyle and disc) violates its normal functional capabilities. It is resisted by the collateral ligaments that unite the articulating parts of the complex. Such movement may damage those ligaments as well as the articular surfaces.

Sliding Action

Passive protective restraint against disarticulation of the temporomandibular joints is provided by the suspensory effect of the two temporomandibular ligaments. The outer oblique fibers of these ligaments restrict dropping of the mandible inferiorly during translatory cycles, especially during power strokes. The inner horizontal fibers restrict displacement of the mandible posteriorly during maximum intercuspation. Unilaterally, they also restrain posterior movement of the lateral pole of the pivoting condyle during a lateral excursion of the mandible. Such restraints do not interfere with normal translatory movements, nor do they enter *actively* into such movements. Power for mandibular movement is provided by action of the musculature.

Rotatory Action

Passive protective restraint against sliding movement between the condyle and articular disc is provided by the collateral ligaments that attach the disc to the medial and lateral poles of the condyle. These discal ligaments do not restrain rotatory movements between disc and condyle, nor do they enter *actively* into disc-condyle complex movements.

Throughout translatory cycles, active anterior rotation of the disc is provided by the superior lateral pterygoid muscle through the effect of muscle tonus. During power strokes and maximum intercuspation, this force is augmented by a strong positive anterior traction force created by active contraction of the muscle. No *active* force rotates the articular disc *posteriorly*, except in the forward phase of the translatory cycle when the superior retrodiscal lamina is stretched. At that time, the articular disc is rotated posteriorly. Therefore, the articular disc normally occupies the most anteriorly rotated position on the condyle permitted by the width of the disc space at all times, except during the full forward phase of the translatory cycle. Then, the disc is rotated posteriorly to prevent spontaneous dislocation.

During power strokes and maximum intercuspation, the disc is rotated anteriorly by strong contraction of the superior lateral pterygoid muscle. This satisfactorily compensates for any change in width of the articular disc space caused by altered interarticular pressure. Otherwise, the rotatory force on the disc is mild, being that of muscle tonus.

The chief purpose of these movements in the disc-condyle complex is to supply adequate stability to the joint by ensuring sharp surface contact of the articulating parts at all times. However, the actual determinant of discal position on the condyle at any given time is the width of the articular disc space as determined by interarticular pressure. Muscle action and elastic traction of the superior retrodiscal lamina that opposes such action merely keep the disc space filled.

Chewing Movements

During chewing movements, muscle action is minimal except with power strokes and maximum intercuspation. Protruder action on the condyle is exerted by contraction of the inferior lateral pterygoid muscle. True protruder muscle action on the articular disc is absent, the superior lateral pterygoid muscle remaining inactive during the forward phase of translation. It contracts only in conjunction with strong elevator action to accomplish power strokes and maximum intercuspation. It acts as the holding muscle on the condyle during the return phase of a power stroke and rotates the articular disc anteriorly to furnish adequate joint stability, especially on the biting side.

Biting against resistance reduces interarticular joint pressure ipsilaterally and, thus, widens the articular disc space. This occurs only during the return phase of a translatory cycle, the exact site being determined by the size and location of the object against which the biting force is directed. The influence on joint pressure due to biting resistance depends on the size and consistency of the object and the speed and power of muscle action.

As the teeth come into contact, the articular disc space on the biting side narrows. At initial contact, there is a momentary decrease in elevator muscle activity (the so-called silent period), presumably due to the inhibitory effect of stimulated periodontal mechanoreceptors. This is followed by marked contraction of the elevator muscles, which brings the teeth into maximum intercuspation. At this point, interarticular pressure is maximal and the articular disc space is minimal, the articular disc being centered with its thinnest central portion between condyle and eminence.

As the dentition takes over the task of stability, the biting force is arrested, and the elevator and superior lateral pterygoid muscles relax back to muscle tonus. In this resting closed position, the articular disc space widens slightly, and muscle tonus in the superior lateral pterygoid muscle rotates a slightly thicker portion of disc anteriorly to maintain sharp contact of the articulating parts.

It should be noted that actual chewing is not defined as precisely as this description would indicate. Many variations of this pattern occur. Although some chewing strokes do end in maximum intercuspation, many do not reach even initial tooth contact, much less full occlusion. The distribution of food between the two sides alters the pattern. Incising and grinding are done differently. The degree of lateral movement utilized with chewing also varies the pattern.

Swallowing involves joint action also. Although it has been thought that swallowing is accompanied by full occlusion of the teeth, it is known that this occurs only with swallowing solid foods. Liquids and automatic swallowing of saliva do not produce this effect.[3] If there is tooth contact at all, it is very light and induces inhibitory influence on elevator muscles due to stimulation of periodontal receptors.

Bruxism, however, is quite a different matter. Whether it is clenching the teeth in firm maximum intercuspation or combined with some movement, bruxism does bring into play similar forces, as described above, which require considerable muscle action and induce alteration of interarticular pressure. This throws a great burden of stress on the joints that may constitute overloading. Also, the demand for rotatory movement in the disc-condyle complex is increased.

STRUCTURAL HARMONY BETWEEN COMPONENTS OF MASTICATORY APPARATUS

Morphologic variation in temporomandibular joints is normal. Condyles and articular eminences vary in size and shape. This is true also of the location of the condyle within the articular fossa. Considerable variation in gross condylar position may be observed in joints that fulfill the criteria of known standards of normal. The important issue is not *morphology* so much as *compatibility* of the parts with each other. This can be summarized as follows:

1. Each temporomandibular joint should present articular surfaces that are compatible in size and shape so that they work in harmony with each other.

2. The two joints should be reasonably compatible with each other bilaterally.

3. The joints should be structurally compatible with the oral structures, particularly the dentition.

Articular Eminence

The most significant structural variant has to do with the inclination of the posterior slope of the articular eminence.[1] Most joints have an inclination of 30 to 60 degrees from the Frankfurt horizontal. Those with inclinations of considerably less are referred to as *flat joints* (Fig 5–1). Those with considerably steeper articular eminences are referred to as *steep joints* (Fig 5–2).

The inclination of the articular eminence relates importantly to disc-condyle complex functioning during translatory movements. Since rotation of the disc on the condyle is necessary to maintain surface-to-surface contact between the disc-condyle complex and the articular eminence during translatory cycles, the flatter the joint, the less the amount of such rotation required. Conversely, the steeper the articular eminence, the greater the rotation of the disc during translation (see Fig 3–6). Very steep joints present the disc-condyle complexes with an extremely difficult task of executing smooth silent translatory cycles, especially if movements are rapid. Such joints, therefore, predispose to discal interference during normal cyclic movements. Also, very steep joints predispose to subluxation with overextended opening because of the necessary posterior rotation of

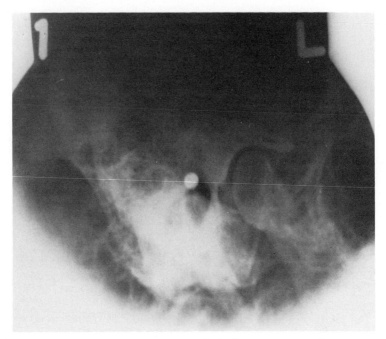

Fig 5-1.—Radiograph illustrates a relatively flat temporomandibular joint. The inclination of the articular eminence is about 24 degrees from the horizontal supra-articular crest.

the articular disc on the condyle required to execute translatory cycles.

The angle of the articular eminence is important during maximum intercuspation if the dentition does not provide adequate stabilizing anchorage when the teeth are fully occluded. In such situations, the steeper the inclination of the articular eminence, the more likely is the disc-condyle complex to slide posteriorly during maximum intercuspation. This increases the burden on the lateral pterygoid muscle to hold the condyle as well as the danger of damage to the inner horizontal fibers of the temporomandibular ligament.

The inclination of the articular eminence also gives information on the relationship between joint morphology, muscle action, and the dentition and oral structures. Very flat joints are more expansive anteroposteriorly. The difference between the mediolateral and anteroposterior diameters of the condyle is less pronounced. The musculature appears to function very well with a minimum of sensory guidance from dental and oral structures, which habitually have more lateral movement in chewing. Compatible oral structures include more expansive dental arches, flatter palate, less over-

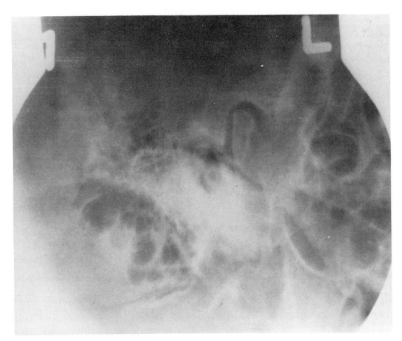

Fig 5–2.—Radiograph illustrates a relatively steep temporomandibular joint. The inclination of the articular eminence is about 70 degrees from the horizontal supra-articular crest.

bite, more shallow fossae, and lower cusps. Such joints present considerable latitude in the occlusal relationship of the teeth in that they function well in an occlusal area, rather than in a precise occlusal position. A "tight" occlusal position actually may induce discomfort and provoke a high degree of oral consciousness.

Very steep joints are usually more compact anteroposteriorly. The difference between the mediolateral and anteroposterior diameters of the condyle is more pronounced. This causes the pivoting condyle during lateral excursions to undergo a greater shift of the vertical axis toward the lateral pole. But considerably less lateral movement is employed habitually in chewing. The musculature appears to depend more heavily on sensory and proprioceptive guidance as the occlusal position is reached. The compatible oral structures include more constricted dental arches, a higher palatal vault, and an interlocking type of dentition with considerable overbite, deeper fossae, and more prominent cusps. Such joints tolerate very little latitude in the occlusal relationship of the teeth and function best with a positive precise occlusal position. In the absence of such a position, considerable oral consciousness may develop, and the patient may complain, "I have lost my bite."

It should be noted that these morphologic relationships are evident only with extremely steep and flat joints. These relationships are not sufficiently pronounced to have clinical significance in most subjects who have an articular eminence inclination between 30 and 60 degrees from horizontal.

Bilateral Compatibility

It is important that the joints be bilaterally compatible with each other. When the difference between the inclination of the articular eminences is considerable, difficulties due to lack of structural harmony may be serious. Other incompatible differences may result from lack of uniform development. Some problems result from the effects of trauma; some are problems of growth, such as hyperplasia of the condyle.

FUNCTIONAL HARMONY BETWEEN MUSCULATURE AND DENTITION

The craniomandibular articulation is unique in one respect: it must reckon with forces incidental to the occlusion of teeth. This is in addition to the forces initiated by muscle action against resistance. It has to do with forces generated by the meshing of inclined planes that comprise the occluding surfaces of teeth, i.e., the forces resulting from maximum intercuspation.[1]

The gross position of the disc-condyle complex relative to the temporal facet at any given time throughout empty-mouth translatory cycles is determined by muscle action. The influence of the teeth is minimal, being largely inhibitory on muscle action as a result of stimulation of periodontal mechanoreceptors.

Power strokes introduce another force that alters the postural relationship between disc-condyle complex and articular eminence. This, however, is resolved by the time the teeth come into contact. Therefore, the unclenched closed position of the joint represents a relationship between the articulating parts that is the product of muscle action. By a combination of conditioned habit patterns, reflex activity, proprioceptive and sensory guidance (including that of the periodontal ligaments), and volition, the position of the disc-condyle complex relative to the articular eminence as the teeth come into contact is determined by muscle action.

As the inclined planes of the occluding teeth come under biting stress supplied by the elevator muscles, a new and irresistible force becomes the final determinant of disc-condyle complex position. This supercedes the effect of muscle action. This force occurs suddenly as the teeth reach maximum intercuspation and disappears just as rapidly when the musculature relaxes following full occlusion of the teeth. The clenched, occluded position of the joint represents a relationship between the articulating parts that is the product of tooth form and position.

The act of maximum intercuspation, therefore, causes a rapid shift of postural forces from muscle action to tooth form and back to muscle action. *This takes place every time the teeth are fully occluded*. It should be obvious that any gross shifting of disc-condyle complex position by these changing forces would be conflictory and, therefore, incompatible with normal joint functioning.

Functional harmony between the masticatory muscles and the dentition, therefore, is present when the muscle-determined position of the disc-condyle complex (which represents the closed unclenched relationship of the joint) is not altered by forces generated by maximum intercuspation of the teeth (the closed clenched relationship of the joint).

Functional Incompatibility

Lack of functional harmony between the muscles and dentition may induce a variety of deleterious effects. When frictional resistance anchors the articular disc, gross movement of the condyle may induce damaging changes in the articular surfaces. Those surfaces in contact when the joint is closed are the ones that bear the burden of stress. Deleterious change causes loss of smoothness of these surfaces. This, in turn, adds to the anchoring effect of the frictional pressure, thus intensifying the possible abuse.

Because of the location of the articular eminence relative to the disc-condyle complex in the closed-joint position, gross movement of the condyle anteriorly while the disc is anchored by friction against the eminence may be damaging to the disc. Such movement of the condyle may also overload the discal collateral ligaments and, thus, permit condylar encroachment upon the thicker anterior portion of articular disc. Such damage may compromise the effectiveness of the articular disc in stabilizing the joint during the forward phase of translatory movement. Deleterious changes affecting the temporal articular surface at the closed-joint position predispose to sticking of the articular disc after maximum intercuspation and hanging of the disc as maximum intercuspation is reached at the end of power strokes.

Initially, posterior displacement of the disc-condyle complex is resisted by the lateral pterygoid muscle, thus inducing muscle effects. Subsequently, it is resisted by the inner horizontal fibers of the temporomandibular ligament. As the articular disc is immobilized against the temporal articular surface by friction, overloading of the discal ligaments may cause deterioration or elongation. This may permit condylar encroachment upon the thicker posterior portion of the disc. Deleterious change in that portion of the disc reduces its effectiveness in stabilizing the joint during power strokes and maximum intercuspation. Elongation of the discal ligaments and inner horizontal fibers of the temporomandibular ligament may also permit condylar encroachment upon the retrodiscal structures.

Posterior overclosure occurs when occlusal support in the molar area is insufficient to prevent movement of the mandible during maximum intercuspation. If the remaining teeth provide sufficient anchorage to prevent movement of the mandible posteriorly, a fulcrum forward to the molar area is established. This causes the direction of force and movement of the condyle to be upward and forward, which may result in overloading against the articular eminence. If, however, the remaining teeth do not so anchor the occlusion, the disc-condyle complex is displaced posteriorly.

If displacement causes either of the discal ligaments to undergo deterioration, elongation, or detachment sufficient to impair its primary function of ensuring hinge movement in the disc-condyle complex, normal functioning may be disrupted throughout translatory cycles, especially in power strokes and maximum intercuspation. This would predispose to disc-interference disorders.

If the functional incompatibility results from recent occlusal change, structural damage to the joint is less likely to occur. Rather, the effects are predominantly muscular. Since such disharmony would constitute a recent environmental change, the altered proprioceptive and sensory input would be more likely to initiate the protective mechanism of muscle splinting. Such an effect, if protracted, may induce muscle spasm activity.

The various effects of functional disharmony between the masticatory muscles and the dentition relate to the closed relationship of the joint— unclenched to clenched occluded position. These effects do not occur when the teeth are separated or very lightly occluded. It is maximum intercuspation, whether due to power strokes and chewing movements or to bruxism, that activates the disharmony.

CLINICAL SYMPTOMS OF TEMPOROMANDIBULAR DISORDERS

Lack of structural or functional harmony between components of the masticatory apparatus may lead to symptoms. Masticatory symptoms may be classified as masticatory pains and masticatory dysfunctions. Different temporomandibular disorders are recognized and identified by combinations of these symptoms.

Masticatory Pains

Masticatory pains are "chewing pains" that have their source in and emanate from the masticatory muscles (myalgia) or temporomandibular joints (arthralgia). This term is not intended to include chewing pains of purely dental or oral origin. Nor should the term be used to include referred pains and nonspastic myofascial pain syndromes. All masticatory pains are of the deep somatic category and have characteristics of the musculoskeletal type.[2]

MASTICATORY MYALGIA.—Pains arising from masticatory muscles have myogenous characteristics. They relate to the demands of function and can be elicited or aggravated by manual palpation or functional manipulation. They may be classified clinically as
1. Muscle splinting pain
2. Muscle spasm pain
3. Muscle inflammation pain
Transitional phases between these types of myalgia may make precise identification difficult, if not impossible.

TEMPOROMANDIBULAR ARTHRALGIA.—Arthralgic pain emanates from the pain-sensitive structures of the temporomandibular joint and usually are predominantly inflammatory in type. They relate to the demands of function and can be elicited or aggravated by manual palpation or functional manipulation. Temporomandibular arthralgia may be classified according to the structure from which it arises as
1. Disc attachment pain
2. Retrodiscal pain
3. Capsular pain
4. Arthropathy pain

Masticatory Dysfunctions

Symptoms of masticatory dysfunction arise as a result of derangements of the masticatory muscles and/or the joints proper. They may be classified as restriction of mandibular movement, interference during mandibular movement, and acute malocclusion.

RESTRICTION OF MANDIBULAR MOVEMENT.—Normally, the masticatory apparatus should function in a way that permits opening of the mouth sufficiently to meet all the requirements for incising and masticating food. Protrusive movement should be sufficient to bring the incisal edges of the teeth together. Lateral movement should permit bringing the upper and lower buccal cusps together. Mandibular movements should be bilaterally symmetric. There should be no appreciable deflection of the midline incisal path during opening or protrusion.

INTERFERENCE DURING MANDIBULAR MOVEMENT.—Interference during mandibular movement may be expressed as

1. Abnormal sensations, such as rubbing, binding, or catching
2. Abnormal sounds, such as discrete clicking, popping, or snapping as well as more continuous grating noise
3. Abnormal movements (irregular, jerky) and deviations of the midline incisal path during opening-closing efforts

ACUTE MALOCCLUSION.—Acute malocclusion is that of recent origin and of which the subject is acutely aware. It may be induced by abnormal muscle action or by changes within the joint proper.

STANDARDS OF NORMAL FOR JUDGING MASTICATORY SYSTEM

The initial step in the clinical management of temporomandibular disorders should be to ascertain that the complaint is, indeed, of masticatory nature. This judgment rests on applying standards of normal.[1]

Clinical Standards of Normal

Normally, the masticatory apparatus should present:

1. Freedom from pain that arises in and emanates from the temporomandibular joints or the muscles of mastication.

2. Mandibular movements that are adequate in amplitude, are symmetric bilaterally, and are not deflected during opening or protruding.

3. Freedom from abnormal sensations, noises, and movements during normal mandibular functioning.

4. Structural harmony between components of the masticatory apparatus.

5. Functional harmony between the unclenched and clenched occluded positions.

Radiographic Standards of Normal

If radiographic evidence is needed for confirmation, one should have access to a series of superimposable joint films made in the following positions: (1) unclenched closed position, (2) clenched occluded position, (3) lateral excursion to the opposite side, and (4) maximum unstrained opening

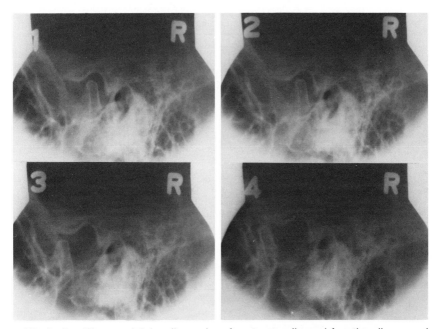

Fig 5–3.—Transparietal radiographs of a structurally and functionally normal temporomandibular joint: *1,* unclenched, closed position of the joint; *2,* clenched, occluded position of the joint (maximum intercuspation); *3,* lateral excursion to the opposite side; *4,* maximum unstrained open position. Within the limitations imposed by flat-plate radiography, the osseous surfaces appear to be well defined, smooth, and rounded in contour; the articular disc space is of sufficient width to accommodate a functioning disc; the condyle in unclenched and clenched occluded positions exactly superimpose; in lateral excursion the condyle reaches the crest of the articular eminence; in open position the condyle movement exceeds that of lateral excursion.

(Fig 5–3). Normal temporomandibular joints should present the following features:

1. The subarticular osseous surfaces should be well defined, smooth, and rounded in contour.

2. The articular disc spaces should be of sufficient width to accommodate functioning articular discs.

3. The condyles in unclenched and clenched occluded positions should exactly superimpose. (Very flat joints may show slight discrepancy.)

4. The condyle position in lateral excursion to the opposite side should reach the crest of the articular eminence.

5. The condyle position in maximum open position should exceed that of lateral excursion to the opposite side.

6. The joints should be bilaterally symmetric structurally.

7. The joints should present bilaterally symmetric condylar movements in opening and lateral excursion to the opposite side.

REFERENCES

1. Bell W.E.: *Temporomandibular Joint Disease*. Dallas, Egan Company Press, 1960, pp. 14–15, 16–18, 40.
2. Bell W.E.: *Orofacial Pains, Differential Diagnosis*, ed. 2. Chicago, Year Book Medical Publishers. 1979.
3. Dubner R., Sessle B.J., Storey A.T.: *The Neural Basis of Oral and Facial Function*. New York, Plenum Press, 1978, pp. 360–362.

6 / Masticatory Pain Symptoms

PAIN is the most important of the various masticatory symptoms, not because it is the most serious or the most frequent, but because it is the symptom that causes the patient the greatest concern and for which he most frequently seeks treatment. Pain, therefore, is the primary issue in the management of temporomandibular disorders. It is the symptom by which most patients judge the results of treatment. It deserves first consideration in the handling of such complaints.

By definition, *masticatory pain* is discomfort about the face and mouth induced by chewing and other jaw use, but independent of local disease involving the teeth and mouth. Masticatory pain has its source in temporomandibular joints and/or masticatory muscles and, therefore, is related directly to masticatory function.[3] It does not include "chewing pains" of dental or pharyngeal origin, pains referred to the joint area, or *nonspastic* myofascial pain syndromes that cause referred pain felt elsewhere. The identification of pain as a valid masticatory symptom hinges on its source: it emanates from the joints or muscles that power the joints and relates to masticatory function.

The *site of pain* (where it is felt) is not necessarily the true *source of pain* (where it actually stems from). Pain arising in another structure may be felt in the masticatory apparatus and may seem to be related to masticatory function. For example, sternocleidomastoid muscle pain may be referred to the temporomandibular joint area. The very first judgment that should be made on pain as a masticatory symptom is whether or not it actually does have its source in temporomandibular joints or masticatory muscles.

Unfortunately, patients, and too frequently their doctors, have insufficient understanding of pain behavior. Pain tends to generate emotional response that is disproportionate to its true significance. If an aura of mystery exists as to the source of pain or its cause, considerable fear may be generated that, in turn, intensifies the pain. Thus, a vicious cycle may develop that induces symptoms bearing little relationship to the initiating cause. To manage pain complaints better, it is necessary to understand some of the mechanisms of pain.

PAIN MODULATION

The time-honored concept of pain behavior is that noxious stimulation of peripheral structures provokes neural impulses that are conducted to the CNS, where they are perceived and reacted to. The reaction is thought to be influenced by such factors as prior conditioning, the emotional significance of the discomfort to the individual, and the general physical and emotional state of the individual at that particular time. This is the *perception-reaction concept* of pain behavior.

In recent years, this understanding of pain behavior has been replaced by the *pain modulation concept*. By pain modulation is meant that the neural impulses generated by noxious stimulation are altered (modulated) prior to being perceived and reacted to. Such modulation is accomplished by peripheral and central inhibitory and excitatory mechanisms operating prior to the noxious stimulation as well as in response to the stimulus. The effect of all modulating factors on the neural impulses is accomplished prior to being perceived. Indeed, the perception of pain is but a facet of the total reaction to those modulated impulses. Thus, when pain is perceived, all factors, including mentation and physical influences, have had their effect already. The suffering itself becomes a continuing modulating influence on the pain. This concept of pain modulation is more consistent with known neurophysiologic facts than the older perception-reaction concept, which failed to explain some features of clinical pain behavior.

Gate-Control Theory of Pain Modulation

The mechanisms by which pain impulses are modulated are in part theoretical. The gate-control theory proposed by Melzack and Wall in 1965 presented a model to help visualize the neural mechanisms involved.[16] This theory has since been expanded.[5] Among neurophysiologists, considerable difference of opinion exists as to the validity of the whole theory. In 1978, Wall reexamined the theory in light of continuing neurophysiologic investigation.[25]

Certain facts have emerged:

1. Intermittent mild stimulation of cutaneous sensory nerves exerts an inhibitory influence on pain.[12, 15, 21] This forms the basis for various treatment modalities such as massage, analgesic balms, vibration, thermal applications, vapocoolants, hydrotherapy, and counterirritation. The recent development of transcutaneous electrical nerve stimulation (so-called TENS units) for the symptomatic relief of pain is based on the inhibitory effect of cutaneous stimulation.

2. The stimulation of specific sites on the body surface exerts a marked

inhibitory influence on pain. These acupoints have been known to the Chinese for many years. Their validity in pain control has been verified by numerous researchers. It has been determined that acuanalgesia induced by the stimulation of such sites is arrested when a local anesthetic is injected into the acupoint being stimulated.[9] It is interesting to note that transcutaneous stimulation applied to acupoints increases its analgesic effect.[19, 20]

3. Pain is increased by certain peripheral and central factors.[16] Hyperemia and inflammation of peripheral tissues reduces the inhibitory influence of the body on pain perception. It is thought that increased small afferent nociceptive fiber activity accounts for this effect. The duration of pain causes it to increase in severity, despite no added peripheral noxious input. It has been thought that this effect is due to the adaptation of thicker nociceptive fibers to noxious stimulation, thereby reducing their inhibitory influence on the pain impulses.

Endogenous Antinociceptive Influence

The recent discovery of endogenous opioids that appear to act as inhibitory neurotransmitters on nociceptive pathways has opened a door to pain behavior at a molecular level. Endorphin (endogenous morphine) in the cerebrospinal fluid (CSF) exerts a definite analgesic effect that is reversible by naloxone, a known morphine antagonist. Endorphins are protein molecules composed of chains of amino acids (peptides). They are secreted by brain tissue into the CSF and by the pituitary gland into the bloodstream. The endorphin level in the CSF is measurable.[22, 24]

Other factors on a molecular level are known to influence pain modulation. Substance P appears to be released from small-diameter primary nociceptive afferents involved in pain transmission. This substance P appears to act as an excitatory transmitter that facilitates pain impulses. Its release is suppressed by β-endorphin as well as by morphine. The suppressive effect is reversed by naloxone.[11] Although large doses of substance P combined with naloxone produce hyperalgesia, tiny doses cause an analgesic effect instead. It is thought, therefore, that small amounts of substance P may release endorphins, whereas larger amounts excite neural activity in nociceptive pathways.[8, 10]

Certain information concerning pain modulation has evolved:

1. Placebo has a therapeutic inhibitory influence on pathologic pain, reducing the pain level by 30% or more.[2] Distraction of the subject's attention also has a therapeutic inhibitory effect as is witnessed by hypnotic suggestion and such techniques as "white sound." Although CSF endorphin level appears not to be increased by hypnosis, it is apparently an integral part of the placebo effect.[13]

2. Endorphin level decreases with the duration of pain and, therefore, relates importantly to chronic pain syndromes.[1, 14, 22]

3. Endorphin level is increased by acupuncture and electroanalgesia. These pain inhibitory effects are reversible by naloxone.[18, 19] Cerebrospinal fluid endorphin does not appear to be increased by transcutaneous electrical nerve stimulation, however, unless it is applied at acupoints.[20] Nevertheless, such stimulation does inhibit pain conduction by some other mechanism, presumably the stimulation of the thicker cutaneous nociceptive afferents, as proposed by the gate-control theory.

Other emerging techniques of pain control should attract sufficient scientific investigation to determine their validity and neurophysiologic foundation, if any. So-called applied kinesiology is one technique that has many advocates on a clinical level.[7] Another technique is osteopathic manipulation or chiropractic adjustment of the cranial bones. Serious controlled investigation of these modalities is warranted.

Another strange technique is auricular diagnosis. French and Chinese acupuncturists claim that a somatotopic mapping of the body is represented in the external ear. Sites of increased electrical conductivity and heightened tenderness that identify the location of pathologic conditions elsewhere in the body are said to be present in the external ear tissues. Difficult as it may be to understand, a recent testing of this form of diagnosis in a group of 40 patients with known musculoskeletal pain indicated auricular diagnosis to be accurate in the range of 70%.[17]

SECONDARY EFFECTS OF DEEP PAIN

Another pain mechanism that has clinical importance, both diagnostically and therapeutically, has to do with secondary effects of deep pain input. Unfortunately, the neurophysiologic mechanisms are obscure and poorly understood. The clinical behavior of these effects, however, is well known.[6] Secondary effects induced by deep pain include (1) referred pain with, and without, secondary hyperalgesia, (2) local autonomic effects, and (3) skeletal muscle effects.

In general, these effects occur as a CNS phenomenon. They probably result from the convergence of impulses conducted by primary afferent neurons onto other interneurons that ordinarily would not be stimulated. Continued deep-pain input appears to cause hyperexcitability of such neurons. These phenomena are referred to as *central excitatory effects*.

Several clinical features of these secondary effects are known:

1. They appear to require continuity of deep-pain input. Some effects, such as referred pain, remain wholly dependent on the primary pain input and disappear when the primary pain is arrested, even temporarily, as with

local analgesic blocking. Some effects, such as secondary hyperalgesia and local autonomic effects, are dependent on the primary pain but may persist for a while after the primary initiating pain ceases. If secondary muscle contraction develops into a cycling muscle spasm, it becomes independent of the initiating pain and behaves instead as a new deep-pain source with the same potentiality of inducing other secondary effects as deep pain elsewhere. Intermittent input does not seem to induce secondary central excitatory effects. The greater the severity and duration, the greater the likelihood that secondary effects will occur.

2. Secondary effects of deep-pain input occur in otherwise *normal* structures. The sites where such effects are seen should be quite innocent and therapy directed toward them is not effective, except for cycling myospasms.

3. The primary-pain input may or may not be felt on a conscious level. If the primary pain is silent, the secondary pain may be mistaken for the true source of pain.

4. Secondary effects are most likely to occur in peripheral structures innervated by other fibers of the same major nerve. If trigeminal secondary effects are expressed in adjacent divisions of the nerve that mediates the input, the effects follow a vertical pattern consistent with the location of sensory nerve cell bodies in the trigeminal nucleus.[4] If structures innervated by a different neural segment become involved, the secondary effects occur predominately in a cephalad direction.[6] Ordinarily, trigeminal pain input does not induce secondary effects outside the vast trigeminal region.

Referred Pains

Heterotopic pain is that which is felt in an area other than the true site of origin. This may occur for different reasons, namely:

1. All pains of psychogenic origin are felt peripherally.

2. Pains arising from structures of the CNS are felt peripherally, those coming from intracranial pain-sensitive structures on or above the tentorium cerebelli being felt in the trigeminal distribution.

3. Some peripheral pains, such as those of deep visceral origin, may be so diffuse in quality that the subject misinterprets their source and feels them in a different location.

4. Noxious stimulation of a sensory nerve trunk (such as dorsal root irritation) and pain arising as a result of peripheral neuropathy (such as neuritis or neuralgia) may be felt as superficial pain projected along the peripheral distribution of that nerve, thus following dermatome mapping accurately enough that the site of pain may be sufficient to identify its true source.

5. Noxious stimulation of a motor nerve trunk (such as ventral root irritation) may cause pain that is felt diffusely in the musculature innervated by that nerve. Such pain is sensed more deeply in the body structures and therefore has little relationship to dermatome geography.

6. True referred pain occurs as a central excitatory effect and, therefore, is a CNS phenomenon in response to continuous noxious deep-pain input.

True referred pain frequently complicates masticatory pain symptoms and therefore should be understood and differentiated clinically from other heterotopic pains. *It requires CNS synapse.* The primary pain responsible for the condition is of deep origin and is mediated in the usual way to the trigeminal nucleus. There the transfer is made (presumably as the result of convergence) in such a way that it is felt as coming from a different site. The *primary pain* is the true source of the complaint; the *secondary pain* is felt in the referred pain site. Provocation of the primary pain site initiates or aggravates both primary and secondary pains; provocation of the secondary pain site does nothing. Analgesic blocking of the pathway that mediates the primary pain arrests both primary and secondary pains; blocking the pathway that subserves the secondary pain site arrests neither pain.

SECONDARY HYPERALGESIA.—Referred pains may or may not be accompanied by areas of secondary hyperalgesia located superficially or deeply in the body structures. Hyperalgesia is defined as excessive sensitivity or sensibility to stimulation (provocation). It may be primary or secondary. *Primary hyperalgesia* results from local cause that has lowered the pain threshold of the structures that hurt. In *secondary hyperalgesia,* no local cause exists for the condition. Pain threshold in the area is essentially normal. It occurs in conjunction with the phenomenon of referred pain and is a true central excitatory effect. Although the hypersensitivity is of the secondary type, a minor portion may be due to primary hyperalgesia, as evidenced by the presence of a small hyperemic zone of axon reflex flare.[6]

Secondary hyperalgesia follows the same general rules that apply to other central excitatory effects, except that it may persist for a while after the primary pain ceases. The area of hypersensitivity may be situated on the surface, or it may occur more deeply in the tissues. Superficial secondary hyperalgesia is felt as *excessive sensitivity to touch.* As such, it usually presents no diagnostic problem. But, if located deeply, it is felt as *tenderness to palpation* and may be confused with other primary pain sources, such as spasm or inflammation of muscle tissue. It is important to be able to differentiate deep secondary hyperalgesia from a true primary-pain source. This may be done by analgesic blocking which completely arrests primary pain but only partially reduces the discomfort of secondary hyperalgesia.

Autonomic Effects

Localized autonomic effects may occur as a central excitatory effect induced by deep-pain input. These effects include color changes, temperature changes, puffy swelling of the eyelids or other loose cutaneous tissue, injection of the conjunctiva, lacrimation, nasal secretion, and nasal congestion. Such effects may be mistaken for allergic rhinitis or acute sinusitis. Although dependent on the continuity of deep-pain input, such symptoms tend to persist for a while after the primary pain ceases.

Muscle Effects

Deep-pain input may cause certain effects in the skeletal muscles as a result of central hyperexcitability. Such effects are predominantly contractile and tend to induce myospasm. If myospasm persists long enough to become painful, a cycling myospasm may develop and remain as a separate clinical entity indefinitely—as a self-perpetuating, pain-dysfunction syndrome.

Muscle effects occur especially in muscles innervated by the same neural segment that mediates the initiating primary pain. Therefore, the muscles innervated by the trigeminal nerve (i.e., the masticatory muscles plus the mylohyoid, anterior digastric, tensor palati, and tensor tympani muscles) are the ones affected by pain from the vast trigeminal region. Since effects of central hyperexcitability occur almost exclusively in a cephalad direction (when extrasegmental reference occurs), other deep-pain sources of facial and cervical origin also may cause muscle effects in trigeminal innervated muscles.

Although muscle effects due to central excitation are usually contractile, it appears from clinical evidence that nonspastic myofascial pain syndromes may be initiated in like manner. Such syndromes may also persist quite independently of the initiating deep-pain input. When this occurs, the referred pain that characterizes nonspastic myofascial pain syndromes often is felt at or near the site of the initiating primary-pain source.

MYOFASCIAL TRIGGERS.—Pain of myofascial origin arises from so-called myofascial triggers located within the muscle or its tendinous attachments. Such trigger points, when stimulated by normal functional activities, cause referred pain that is felt elsewhere outside the muscle proper. These trigger sites, however, are locally tender to manual palpation, with or without simultaneous reference of pain. The patient may be wholly unaware of the muscular source of the pain and may think the site of pain represents the cause of his complaint. The involved muscle(s) may otherwise be quite normal. The zones of reference for such trigger points have been well charted by Travell and Rinzler.[23] That such triggers do exist and cause referred pain is unmistakable, even though the mechanism involved is not clear. Analgesic blocking of such trigger points arrests the reference of pain.

Myofascial pains are frequently associated with myospastic activity. When involving the masticatory muscles, the condition is popularly known as a myofascial pain-dysfunction (MPD) syndrome. No doubt, much of the referred pain that characterizes this temporomandibular disorder arises from myofascial triggers. It should be understood, however, that some myofascial pain syndromes do not have a component of muscle spasm. These are the ones that a patient may be wholly unaware of. Since the pain of nonspastic myofascial pain syndromes is referred outside the muscle, and since there is no muscle dysfunction present, such conditions do not constitute a masticatory muscle *complaint* and, therefore, comprise no temporomandibular disorder. Such conditions do sometimes become spastic, and when this occurs, an acute muscle disorder becomes evident.

DIFFERENTIAL CHARACTERISTICS OF PAIN

Different facial pain syndromes are identified best by comparing their clinical characteristics. Different pain syndromes may behave much alike in many respects and are best identified by their differences than by their similarities. The initial step in precise pain identification is recognition of which general pain category is represented by the particular pain complaint under investigation.[4]

Category Recognition

Orofacial pains may be categorized into four main groups, namely, superficial somatic pain, deep somatic and visceral pain, neurogenous pain, and psychogenic pain. The first two pertain to pains that result from noxious stimulation of body structures innervated by normal neural components, the first arising from superficial structures like the skin and mucogingival tissues, the second arising from deeper body structures and viscera. The third pertains to pain that occurs as a result of abnormality in the neural system (neuropathy). The fourth includes pains that result from certain psychic influences and conditions.

The differential clinical characteristics of superficial, deep, and neurogenous pain categories are listed in Table 6–1. Psychogenic pains may present clinical characteristics of either of the three categories in the table. Such pains are recognized by departure from usual anatomical location, inadequacy of peripheral cause, and unusual physiologic behavior, namely, (1) they may be multiple and/or bilaterally situated, (2) they may lack ade-

TABLE 6–1.—CATEGORIES OF OROFACIAL PAIN SYNDROMES
(DIFFERENTIAL CLINICAL CHARACTERISTICS)

	SUPERFICIAL PAINS	DEEP PAINS	NEUROGENOUS PAINS
1. Systemic effect of pain	Stimulating	Depressing	Stimulating
2. Subject's ability to localize the pain	Excellent	Poor	Excellent
3. Relationship between site of pain and its true source	Same	May or may not be the same	Not the same (except traumatic neuroma)
4. Response to provocation	Faithful	Not faithful in location	Not faithful (except traumatic neuroma)
5. Effects that may accompany pain	None	Effects of central excitation	Direct neurologic effects
6. Effect of topical anesthetic applied to site of pain	Arrests the pain	None (except accessible visceral mucosa)	None (except accessible superficial triggers)

TABLE 6–2.—CLINICAL CHARACTERISTICS THAT IDENTIFY TYPE OF DEEP SOMATIC AND VISCERAL PAIN

	ODONTOGENOUS PAIN	MUSCULOSKELETAL PAIN	VASCULAR PAIN	VISCERAL PAIN
1. Local etiologic factors chiefly responsible for the syndrome	Oral environmental conditions	Functional abuse of muscles and joints	None (except cranial arteritis)	Inflammation and hyperemia of viscera
2. Local factors that initiate or aggravate the pain	Noxious oral stimuli	Manual palpation or functional manipulation	None (except cranial arteritis)	Pressure or palpation of viscera
3. Dysfunction that may accompany the pain	None	Dysfunction due to muscular or joint causes	None	None
4. Temporal behavior of the pain	Pulpal to periodontal sequence; inflammatory curve	No time frame (unless due to inflammation)	Periodic, recurrent (except cranial arteritis)	Parallels resolution of cause

quate peripheral anatomical input, and (3) their behavior is characterized by changeableness, chronicity, and unusual response to therapy.

Kinds of Deep Pain

The second step in precise pain identification consists of differentiating the several kinds of deep pain. These are odontogenous pain, musculoskeletal pain, vascular pain, and visceral pain.

The different features by which these kinds of deep pain can be recognized clinically are listed in Table 6–2. Pains may not present clearly typical behavioral characteristics, due in part to modulation and to central excitatory effects. This applies especially to deep-pain syndromes. Therefore, a description of its early behavior may reflect more accurately the true clinical characteristics that are typical of a particular pain syndrome.

Kinds of Musculoskeletal Pain

Depending on its source, musculoskeletal pain may be classified as muscle pain, joint pain, soft connective tissue pain, or osseous pain. *Masticatory pains are either muscular or arthralgic.*

MUSCLE PAIN.—Muscle pain is more labile in behavior, being characterized by sudden onset, rapid change, variability, and recurrence. It may be accompanied by some muscular dysfunction, if no more than the inhibitory influence of the pain itself. Muscle pain is usually quite responsive to therapy, unless it is due to inflammation.

Myogenous pain may be due to (1) local cause, such as myositis, in which the dysfunction is due to swelling and stiffness associated with the inflammatory process, (2) muscle splinting, which displays very little dysfunction other than minor resistance to stretch, (3) nonspastic myofascial pain, which shows no structural dysfunction at all, and (4) muscle spasm, which causes dysfunction due to rigidity or shortening of the muscle.

JOINT PAIN.—Joint pain arises only from those joint structures that are innervated by sensory receptors. No pain can arise from the articular surfaces or articular disc proper in the absence of trauma or disease. Arthralgia is more stabile, being characterized by insidious onset, slower change, persistence, and resistance to therapy. Such pains are inflammatory in type. Temporomandibular arthralgia is classified according to the structure that is predominantly involved, namely, disc-attachment pain, retrodiscal pain, capsular pain, and arthropathy pain.

IDENTIFYING CRITERIA FOR MASTICATORY MYALGIA

Rational effective management of masticatory pain of muscle origin requires that the particular kind of myogenous pain be identified, if possible. When the complaint represents a transitional phase between two kinds of muscle pain, it is well to plan therapy based on the more resistant of the two conditions. It is usually possible to recognize the kind of myalgia present by observing certain criteria.

Protective Muscle Splinting

ETIOLOGY.—Muscle splinting is thought to occur in response to afferent input that signals the presence of injury or threat of injury (i.e., a marked change from the usual sensory or proprioceptive input). The history, therefore, should indicate prior injury, change in the oral environment, dental treatment (especially with local anesthesia), increased oral consciousness (e.g., evoked volitional chewing that conflicts with established habitual patterns), or stress-induced bruxism.

SYMPTOMS.—Onset of pain is sudden. It occurs when muscles are contracted. Moderate muscle stiffness and a feeling of muscular weakness usually are present.

MUSCULAR DYSFUNCTION.—Muscle splinting causes slightly increased resistance to passive stretch. Except for the inhibitory influence of pain and the sensation of muscular weakness, little or no structural dysfunction is present.

CLINICAL COURSE.—Muscle splinting disappears when the injury or threat resolves. Abusive use or injudicious therapy may protract the splinting effect. *Protracted splinting may induce muscle spasm.*

Masticatory Myospasm

ETIOLOGY.—Myospasm may occur spontaneously, especially in tense individuals. By way of protracted muscle splinting, many local conditions may induce muscle spasm. These include minor strains, abusive use, bruxism, and muscle fatigue. Myospastic activity may occur with or without a prior stage of nonspastic myofascial pain due to systemic causes such as illness, infection, or emotional stress. It may occur as a side effect of certain medications (e.g., phenothiazines). A frequent cause of masticatory myospasm is a continuous input of deep pain located elsewhere (as a central excitatory effect). This may occur not only as the result of deep trigeminal pain, but also in response to facial, glossopharyngeal, and particularly cervical pain sources. It should be noted that in all cases of cycling muscle spasm, the mere presence of myospastic activity does not indicate its proximate cause or even if a cause persists, since such conditions become self-perpetuating and wholly independent of the initiating cause.

Symptoms.—Sudden onset, with or without prior occurrence, is characteristic. Pain is felt with stretching or contraction of the spastic muscle. Elevator muscle spasm causes pain with opening (due to stretching the muscle) or biting and chewing (due to contracting the muscle). Lateral pterygoid spasm causes pain especially with maximum intercuspation (due to stretching the muscle). Minor discomfort may be elicited by opening against resistance (due to contracting the muscle).

Muscular dysfunction.—Muscle spasm causes structural dysfunction, the type depending on the muscle(s) involved and the kind of spasm (isotonic or isometric). Isotonic spasm shortens the muscle. Therefore, such spasm in elevator muscles causes trismus and deflection of the midline incisal path with opening but not with protrusion. Such spasm of the masseter or temporalis muscle deflects ipsilaterally; medial pterygoid spasm deflects contralaterally. Isotonic spasm of the lateral pterygoid muscle causes acute malocclusion, but no trismus. Isometric spasm induces resistance to stretch and some muscular rigidity. It should be noted that myospasm of elevator muscles may increase the interarticular pressure within the joint sufficiently to induce some discal interference (see chapter 7).

Clinical course.—Cycling myospasm becomes self-perpetuating and therefore tends to persist. If abused or injudiciously treated (especially by excessive exercising), protracted myospasm may become inflammatory and present as masticatory myositis.

Masticatory Myositis

Etiology.—Masticatory myositis may result from any local cause, such as unaccustomed use, abuse, injury, infection, or adjacent disease. It may be secondary to another inflammatory condition due to surgery, trauma, or infection. By way of muscle splinting and protracted myospasm, myositis may result from any and all causes of muscle pain.

Symptoms.—Pain occurs with the muscle at rest and with all use. It parallels the clinical course of the inflammatory process.

Muscular dysfunction.—The stiffness and swelling due to the inflammatory process cause trismus if elevator muscles are involved. Myositis of the lateral pterygoid muscle interferes with normal functioning due to the inhibitory effects of pain, but causes very little structural dysfunction.

CLINICAL COURSE.—The incidence, development, leveling off, and resolution of the condition are timed to the determinants of severity and phase of the inflammatory process.

IDENTIFYING CRITERIA FOR TEMPOROMANDIBULAR ARTHRALGIA

Effective management of temporomandibular arthralgia depends considerably on precise knowledge of the type of pain present and from what structure(s) it emanates. The type of arthralgia usually may be determined by observing certain identifying criteria.

Disc-Attachment Pain

ETIOLOGY.—Pain that emanates from the collateral ligaments that attach the articular disc to the medial and lateral poles of the mandibular condyle occurs as a result of strain on those ligaments as they resist displacement between disc and condyle. Therefore, evidence of discal interference during mandibular movements usually is present (see chap. 7).

SYMPTOMS.—Pain occurs in conjunction with the discal interference present. Momentary pain with or immediately prior to symptoms of discal interference usually is indicative of functional strain on the ligaments. More constant pain that is aggravated by such interference suggests the presence of inflammatory change. If the disc-attachment pain relates intimately to maximum intercuspation, it usually can be reduced by biting against a separator that prevents such intercuspation.

DYSFUNCTION.—Joint dysfunction consists of interference with normal articular disc functioning during mandibular movements, expressed as abnormal sensations, noises, movements, and deviations of the incisal path.

CLINICAL COURSE.—The ligaments are innervated with receptors that may induce a variety of muscle effects (muscle splinting, etc.). Inflamed collateral ligaments may induce capsulitis secondarily. Abusive strains and forces on the ligaments may cause elongation, degenerative change, or detachment, thus disrupting the integrity of the disc-condyle complex and predisposing to greater discal interference (see chap. 7). Such change in the collateral ligaments of the disc-condyle complex is irreversible.

Retrodiscal Pain

ETIOLOGY. — Pain emanating from the retrodiscal tissue is chiefly inflammatory and due to injury inflicted by encroachment of the mandibular condyle. Extrinsic trauma is a frequent cause. But, if the dentition is such that it does not satisfactorily anchor the mandible in maximum intercuspation, abusive strain on the inner horizontal fibers of the temporomandibular ligament may result. This may lead to elongation or degenerative change that permits condylar encroachment on the retrodiscal tissue.

SYMPTOMS. — Retrodiscal pain occurs during maximum intercuspation. It is preventable by biting against a separator that prevents full intercuspation.

DYSFUNCTION. — Retrodiscal swelling and/or excessive intracapsular fluid may displace the condyle in the resting closed position of the joint, thus causing acute malocclusion.

CLINICAL COURSE. — The pain follows an inflammatory pattern if the condition is due to acute extrinsic trauma. Hemarthrosis may predispose to fibrous ankylosis. Degeneration or elongation of the temporomandibular ligament predisposes to chronicity.

Capsular Pain

ETIOLOGY. — Capsular pain is due to synovitis or inflammation of the capsule as the result of (1) trauma, (2) direct extension of inflammation from injured discal collateral ligaments or temporomandibular ligament, (3) arthritis or periarticular inflammation, or (4) abuse to preexistent capsular fibrosis.

SYMPTOMS. — Capsulitis is characterized by palpable tenderness directly over the joint proper. Pain is increased with movements that stretch the capsule. If the capsulitis is due to discal or temporomandibular ligament injury, pain also increases in maximum intercuspation and is decreased by biting against a separator.

DYSFUNCTION. — Including the inhibitory influence of pain, dysfunction due to capsulitis may range from minor restriction of function, noticeable only in extended movements, to immobilization of the joint. Excessive intracapsular fluid may cause acute malocclusion. If the condition is secondary to articular disc interference, inflammatory arthritis, inflamed capsular fibrosis, or periarticular conditions, other dysfunction consistent with such conditons may be observed and no doubt will persist after the capsular inflammation is resolved.

CLINICAL COURSE.—Persistence of capsular inflammation predisposes to capsular fibrosis.

Arthropathy Pain

ETIOLOGY.—The pain is due to (1) inflammatory arthritis or (2) inflammation of adhesions of ankylosis that are injured by abusive chewing movements or other jaw use.

SYMPTOMS.—The pain relates to the kind, degree, duration, and phase of the inflammatory condition present. There is usually some secondary capsulitis present also.

DYSFUNCTION.—Restriction and interference relate to the type of arthropathy present. Intracapsular inflammatory effusion may cause acute malocclusion.

CLINICAL COURSE.—Chronicity is characteristic. If pain is due to inflamed ankylosis, restricted movement will remain after the pain disappears.

POSITIVE IDENTIFICATION OF MASTICATORY PAIN

By comparing their differential clinical characteristics, orofacial pain syndromes may be classified as indicated in Chart 6–1.[4] Myogenous masticatory pains may represent examples of muscle splinting, muscle spasm, or myositis (local muscle soreness). It is to be understood, however, that masticatory myospasm can be a central excitatory effect due to the input of arthralgic pain, providing it is continuous. Intermittent arthralgia does not present this complication.

All masticatory pain is musculoskeletal and of the deep category. Therefore, masticatory pains should present clinical characteristics consistent with deep pain of musculoskeletal type. It is by these characteristics that true masticatory pain can be differentiated from entities such as atypical facial neuralgia (vascular pain), reflex sympathetic dystrophy (visceral pain), glossopharyngeal neuritis (neurogenous pain), and glossopharyngeal neuralgia (neurogenous pain).[4]

It is necessary, however, to ascertain that the pain in question does emanate from the temporomandibular joint or a masticatory muscle. Three criteria are useful in making this judgment:

1. *The pain must relate precisely to mandibular activity*. This determination is made by relating the pain to (1) empty-mouth translatory cycles for opening, protruding, and making lateral excursions, (2) power strokes ending in maximum intercuspation, and (3) clenching the teeth from the unclenched closed position.

CHART 6-1.—CLASSIFICATION OF OROFACIAL PAINS BASED ON THEIR
CLINICAL CHARACTERISTICS

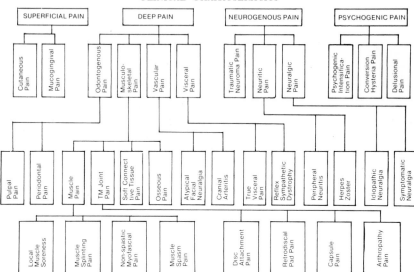

(Reproduced with permission from Bell W.E.: *Orofacial Pains: Differential Diagnosis,* ed. 2. Copyright © 1979 by Year Book Medical Publishers, Inc., Chicago.)

To distinguish mandibular activity from lip, tongue, and throat pains that are elicited incidentally with chewing, swallowing, or talking, the mandible should be stabilized by biting lightly against a small bite block (to immobilize the joints and muscles). Then the lips, tongue, and throat can be manipulated separately from jaw movements to identify pain sources that are only incidental to jaw movement.

2. *The pain is initiated or aggravated by manual palpation or functional manipulation of the joints or masticatory muscles.* Manual palpation should elicit discomfort emanating from that particular structure, providing it is accessible (e.g., the joints proper, the masseter muscle, and the temporalis muscle). The medial pterygoid muscle is not accessible unless the mouth can be opened well. The lateral pterygoid is not accessible to manual palpation at all. Functional manipulation therefore should be employed to identify the presence of pain due to stretching or contracting these muscles.

Manipulation of the lateral pterygoid muscle consists of (1) protruding the jaw against resistance (to contract the muscle) and (2) having the subject bite against a separator (which reduces pain induced by stretching the muscle during maximum intercuspation).

Manipulation of the medial pterygoid muscle consists of (1) opening widely (to stretch the muscle) and (2) having the subject bite against a separator (which *does not* reduce the pain because it does not prevent contraction of the muscle).

3. *Pain provoked by manual palpation or functional manipulation is arrested by analgesic blocking of the structure from which it emanates.* If positive confirmation of the pain source is needed, analgesic blocking can be used. This will differentiate primary pain sources from sites of secondary hyperalgesia (see Figs 9–1 through 9–4). Actively inflamed structures should be avoided. Muscle injections should contain no epinephrine-like vasoconstrictor in order to avoid the vasodilating effect of stimulated sympathetic efferents in muscle tissue. Otherwise, the rules for such injections remain those standard for all injections, namely, (1) achieve asepsis, (2) aspirate before depositing the solution, (3) know the anatomical structures through which the needle passes, and (4) know the solution being used. Usually, injection into the muscles is preferred to injection of the joint proper. If it is necessary to anesthetize the joint, it is done by infiltrating the auriculotemporal nerve at a point just posterior to the neck of the condylar process. Usually a second infiltration is needed just anterior to the joint proper to arrest sensation from the anterior third of the capsule.

It should be noted that local anesthesia about the temporomandibular area also may affect motor fibers of the facial nerve. The resulting eyelid paralysis lasts only for the duration of the anesthesia.

REFERENCES

1. Almay B.G.L., Johansson F., Von Knorring L., et al.: Endorphins in chronic pain: I. Differences in CSF endorphin levels between organic and psychogenic pain syndromes. *Pain* 5:153, 1978.
2. Beecher H.K.: The use of chemical agents in the control of pain, in Knighton R.S., Dumke P.R. (eds.): *Pain, Henry Ford Hospital International Symposium.* Boston, Little, Brown & Co., 1966, pp. 221–239.
3. Bell W.E.: Management of masticatory pain, in Alling C.C. (ed.): *Facial Pain.* Philadelphia, Lea & Febiger, 1968, pp. 191–212.
4. Bell W.E.: *Orofacial Pains, Differential Diagnosis,* ed. 2. Chicago, Year Book Medical Publishers, 1979.
5. Casey K.L., Melzack R.: Neural mechanisms of pain: A conceptual model, in Way E.L. (ed.): *New Concepts in Pain.* Philadelphia, F. A. Davis Co., 1967, pp. 12–31.
6. Dalessio D.J.: *Wolff's Headache and Other Head Pain,* ed. 3. New York, Oxford University Press, 1972.
7. Eversaul G.A.: Applied kinesiology and the treatment of TM dysfunction, in Gelb H. (ed.): *Clinical Management of Head, Neck, and TMJ Pain and Dysfunction.* Philadelphia, W. B. Saunders Co., 1977, pp. 480–506.
8. Frederickson R.C.A., Burgis V., Harrell C.E., et al.: Dual actions of substance

P on nociception: Possible role of endogenous opioids. *Science* 199:1359, 1978.

9. Hannington-Kiff J.G.: *Pain Relief.* Philadelphia, J.B. Lippincott Co., 1974.
10. Henry J.L., Sessle B.J., Lucier G.E., et al.: Effects of substance P on nociceptive and nonnociceptive trigeminal brain stem neurons. *Pain* 8:33, 1980.
11. Jessell T.M., Iverson L.L.: Opiate analgesics inhibit substance P release from rat trigeminal nucleus. *Nature* 268:549, 1977.
12. Kane K., Taub A.: A history of local electrical analgesia. *Pain* 1:125, 1975.
13. Levine J.D., Gordon N.C., Fields H.L.: The role of endorphins in placebo analgesia, in Bonica J.J., Liebeskind J.C., Albe-Fessard D.G. (eds.): *Advances in Pain Research and Therapy.* New York, Raven Press, 1979, vol. 3, pp. 547–551.
14. Lindblom U., Tegner R.: Are the endorphins active in clinical pain states? Narcotic antagonism in chronic pain patients. *Pain* 7:65, 1979.
15. Long D.M., Hagfors N.: Electrical stimulation in the nervous system: The current status of electrical stimulation of the nervous system for relief of pain. *Pain* 1:109, 1975.
16. Melzack R., Wall P.D.: Pain mechanisms: A new theory. *Science* 150:971, 1965.
17. Oleson T.D., Kroening R.J., Bresler D.E.: An experimental evaluation of auricular diagnosis: The somatotopic mapping of musculoskeletal pain at ear acupuncture points. *Pain* 8:217, 1980.
18. Pomerantz B., Cheng R.: Suppression of noxious impulses in single neurons of cat spinal cord by electroacupuncture and its reversal by opiate antagonist naloxone. *Exp. Neurol.* 64:327, 1979.
19. Sjolund B.H., Ericksson M.B.E.: Electroacupuncture and endogenous morphine. *Lancet* 2:1085, 1976.
20 Sjolund B.H., Ericksson M.B.E.: Endorphins and analgesia produced by peripheral conditioning stimulation, in Bonica J.J., Liebeskind J.C., Albe-Fessard D.G. (eds.): *Advances in Pain Research and Therapy.* New York, Raven Press, 1979, vol. 3, pp. 587–592.
21. Sternbach R.H., Ignelzi R.J., Deems L.M., et al.: Transcutaneous electrical analgesia: A follow-up analysis. *Pain* 2:34, 1976.
22. Terenius L.: Endorphins in chronic pain, in Bonica, J.J., Liebeskind J.C., Albe-Fessard D.G. (eds.): *Advances in Pain Research and Therapy.* New York, Raven Press, 1979, vol. 3, pp. 459–471.
23. Travell J., Rinzler S.H.: The myofascial genesis of pain. *Postgrad. Med. J.* 11:425, 1952.
24. Von Knorring L., Almay B.G.L., Johansson F., et al.: Pain perception and endorphin levels in cerebrospinal fluid. *Pain* 5:359, 1978.
25. Wall P.D.: The gate control theory of pain mechanisms: A reexamination and restatement. *Brain* 101:1, 1978.

7 / Masticatory Dysfunction Symptoms

MOST TEMPOROMANDIBULAR COMPLAINTS have a component of dysfunction that is expressed as (1) inability to move the jaw normally, (2) various noises and sensations of interference that occur during jaw movements, or (3) some recent alteration in the way the teeth come together. Effective management of temporomandibular disorders depends on precise identification of the kind of dysfunction present in the complaint, where it is located, and what chiefly is responsible for it.

More specifically, masticatory dysfunction symptoms are classified into three groups, as follows:[1]

1. Restriction of mandibular movement
2. Interference during mandibular movement
3. Acute malocclusion

RESTRICTION OF MANDIBULAR MOVEMENT

The normal range of movement of the mandible is that which is adequate for the purpose intended—mastication and talking. Abnormality in this regard is an individual matter. For a particular individual, restriction of mandibular movement is symptomatic of masticatory dysfunction when it interferes in some way with his usual masticatory activities.

Pseudoankylosis

If mandibular movement becomes restricted for reasons quite independent of the joint proper, the condition is usually classified as *pseudoankylosis*, which may result from a variety of causes.

Cicatricial tissue involving the lips can cause microstomia that restricts mouth opening. This may occur as the result of burns especially. Extensive ulceration of the oral mucosa may cause contractures to form between the maxillary and mandibular arches; this can impose severe limitation on mouth opening (Fig 7–1). Depressed fractures of the zygomatic arch and traumatic displacement of the coronoid process may cause interference with normal mandibular movements. Hypertrophy of the coronoid process reactive to injury also may interfere with jaw functioning. Tumor formation, especially malignant invasion (Figs 7–2 and 7–3), and inflammatory

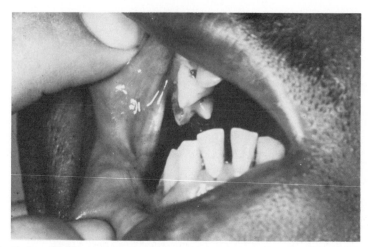

Fig 7–1.—Mouth opening is restricted to 20-mm interincisal distance because of cicatricial contracture in the right buccal mucosa that developed as a result of extensive ulceration from mercurial poisoning.

conditions of the face and jaws (Fig 7–4) may seriously interfere with movements of the mandible.

All such complaints due to pseudoankylosis should be recognized and differentiated from the true temporomandibular disorders, because the treatment is not the same.

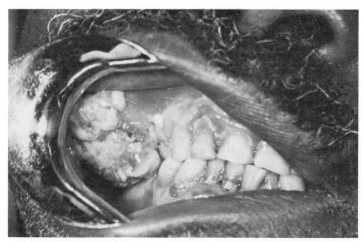

Fig 7–2.—Mouth opening is restricted to a few millimeters due to invasive adenocarcinoma involving the posterior maxillary and mandibular area.

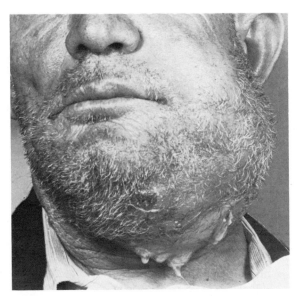

Fig 7-3.—Left temporomandibular joint is immobilized by invasive squamous cell carcinoma.

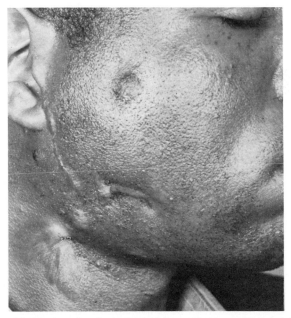

Fig 7-4.—Mouth opening is restricted by actinomycosis involving the right facial, cervical, and masseter muscle area.

True Temporomandibular Restriction of Movement

Restriction of mandibular movement more frequently results from causes related directly to the joint and particularly to the masticatory muscles. Depending on where the cause is located, such limitation of movement is classified as extracapsular, capsular, or intracapsular. It is of considerable diagnostic and therapeutic importance that the location of restraint be identified properly. This can be done by observing certain clinical criteria. Confirmation, if needed, can be done radiographically.

EXTRACAPSULAR RESTRAINT.—Although an occasional nonmasticatory extracapsular cause for restricted jaw movement does occur, the usual cause is a shortened or immobilized elevator muscle due to spasm, inflammation, or contracture.

A shortened elevator muscle restricts mouth opening without appreciably affecting protrusion or lateral excursion. Therefore, the clinical symptoms of myogenous restriction of mandibular movement are:

1. Restricted opening, but fairly normal protrusion and lateral excursion to the opposite side.

2. Deflection of the midline incisal path with opening, but not with protrusion.

3. Pain, if any, increases with opening widely (due to stretching the painful muscle) and with biting (due to contracting the painful muscle).

Deflection of the incisal path is to be distinguished from deviation. *Deflection* refers to a continuing eccentric displacement of the midline incisal path and is symptomatic of restriction of movement. *Deviation* refers to discursive movement that ends in the centered position and is indicative of interference during movement.

When opening is restricted, deflection of the midline incisal path may occur. Shortening of an elevator muscle arrests opening without affecting the capability of the disc-condyle complex to execute translatory movements. Unless inhibited by the effect of pain, protrusive and lateral movements remain normal. But, if an attempt is made to open the mouth more widely, the mandible deflects, thus permitting the teeth to be separated farther. This deflection is due to lateral excursive movement. *The direction that it takes depends on the location of the shortened muscle(s)*. The masseter and temporalis muscles are located lateral to the condyle. A shortened masseter or temporalis muscle does not inhibit freedom of lateral excursion in the opposite joint. Because of such translatory movement in the opposite joint, a shortened masseter or temporalis muscle permits deflection of the midline incisal path ipsilaterally (to the same side). This is not true, however, of the medial pterygoid muscle. Being located medial to the condyle, a shortened medial pterygoid muscle causes translatory movement in the ipsilateral rather than the opposite joint, a movement similar to that of the balancing condyle in a normal lateral excursive movement. The opposite condyle remains seated. Thus, the midline incisal path is deflected contralaterally (to the opposite side). It should be noted, however, that contralateral deflection induced by a shortened medial pterygoid muscle may be observed only if that is the sole muscle involved.

Deflection of the incisal path begins immediately as the restraining effect of a shortened elevator muscle arrests the opening effort. Thus, the point at which obvious deflection commences indicates the degree of shortening of the muscle. Since the deflection itself is due to lateral excursion of the mandible, the amount of deflection is indicative of the degree of lateral excursion that takes place.

Deflection with opening may not occur, or does so very slightly, (1) if the medial pterygoid muscle is involved in conjunction with the masseter or temporalis muscles, (2) if bilateral extracapsular restraint involves both joints, or (3) if the opposite joint is incapable of significant lateral movement.

Deflection with opening can occur, *but it may not do so* if the musculature (usually the opposite temporalis muscle) holds the opposite condyle in sympathetic posture with the affected side. This usually is due to the inhibitory influence of pain. When deflection does not take place, the separation of the teeth is less, and the resultant trismus is relatively greater.

Radiographic confirmation of extracapsular restriction of mandibular movement is done by comparing the condylar position in maximum opening with that of lateral excursion to the opposite side. The condyle position in lateral excursion will appear normal, whereas in the open position it will be considerably less (Fig 7–5).

CAPSULAR RESTRAINTS.—Reduction in the size and flexibility of the capsular ligament imposes limitation on the extent of translatory movement of the disc-condyle complex. Such limitation occurs whether the translatory movement is for opening, protrusion, or lateral excursion, and condylar restriction exists to the same degree for all such movements. When capsular restraint is minor, condylar restriction may be evident in the outer ranges of movement only. The degree of restraint depends on the amount of change in capsular size and flexibility. Capsular restraint of mandibular movement may result from inflammatory swelling of the capsule (capsulitis due to various causes) or to fibrotic contracture of the capsule (capsular fibrosis due to prior capsulitis or scarring from injury or surgery).

The most reliable clinical indication of capsular restraint is that its effect on condylar movement remains exactly the same, whether it is for opening,

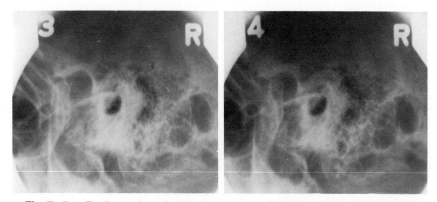

Fig 7–5.—Radiographs of right temporomandibular joint illustrate extracapsular restriction of mandibular movement. *Left,* lateral excursion to the opposite side. *Right,* maximum opening. Note that condylar movement in lateral excursion is within normal limits, while in maximum opening it is less than that of lateral excursion. (From Bell W.E.: Management of temporomandibular joint problems, in Goldman H.M., Gilmore H.W., Royer R.Q., et al. (eds.): *Current Therapy In Dentistry.* St. Louis, C.V. Mosby Co., 1970, vol. 4. Reproduced with permission.)

protrusion, or contralateral excursion. Rotatory opening is not affected, unless inhibited by pain or intracapsular effusion. Therefore, an opening capability of 25 mm (more or less) is present, even though the patient may be reluctant to move the jaw to that extent.

Radiographic confirmation is accurate due to the sameness of the restraining effect on condylar movement in the different positions. It is usually sufficient to compare the open and lateral excursion joint positions. The condyle shadows will exactly superimpose in the two views. In capsular restraint of moderate degree, the condylar position may be just short of the crest of the articular eminence (Fig 7–6).

Capsular restraint due to capsulitis, as a progressive effect of inflammation of the discal collateral ligaments (discitis) or the inner portion of the temporomandibular ligament, may complicate some disc-interference disorders. The pain of such capsulitis is increased with maximum intercuspation and reduced by biting against a separator. Capsular restraint due to capsulitis may also accompany inflammatory arthritis. It is important therapeutically that such restraint be clearly differentiated from extracapsular restrictions due to secondary muscle spasm or other causes.

INTRACAPSULAR RESTRAINTS.—The most frequent cause of intracapsular restriction of mandibular movement is obstruction of the articular disc, which tends to prevent further movement of the condyle. This can occur

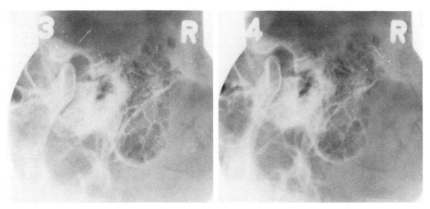

Fig 7–6.—Radiographs of right temporomandibular joint illustrate capsular restriction of mandibular movement. *Left,* lateral excursion to the opposite side. *Right,* maximum opening. Note that condylar movement in lateral excursion is short of the crest of the articular eminence. The restriction in maximum opening is exactly the same. (From Bell W.E.: Management of temporomandibular joint problems, in Goldman H.M., Gilmore H.W., Royer R.Q., et al. (eds.): *Current Therapy In Dentistry.* St. Louis, C.V. Mosby Co., 1970, vol. 4. Reproduced with permission.)

for different reasons, including (1) excessive passive interarticular pressure, (2) structural incompatibility of the articulating parts, (3) impairment of disc-condyle complex function, especially a damaged articular disc in conjunction with dysfunctional discal collateral ligaments, and (4) gross change in the joint due to arthritis. A less frequent but significantly important cause of intracapsular restriction of mandibular movement has to do with blockage of forward translation of the condyle by a dislocated articular disc due to functional displacement[2] or trauma.[4] Fibrous or osseous ankylosis also induces restriction of movement.

Any condition that positively arrests translatory movement within the joint affects all movements—opening, protrusion, and lateral excursions. This accounts for the clinical symptoms, namely:

1. Restriction of opening to the amount permitted by rotatory movement only, plus whatever translatory movement occurs before arrest takes place.

2. Arrested protrusive movement.

3. Arrested contralateral excursive movement.

4. Deflection of the midline incisal path ipsilaterally (toward the symptomatic side) with opening and protrusion.

Deflection of the midline incisal path relates precisely to the point of arrested forward movement of the disc-condyle complex. Some variation in symptoms may occur, especially with disc jamming and protracted anterior functional dislocation as different mandibular movements are examined. These different movements are not identical, and the conditions that cause discal obstruction may vary. This applies especially to the significant difference that exists between empty-mouth movements and power strokes.

It is important therapeutically to differentiate between the different kinds of intracapsular restriction of mandibular movement.

Disc Jamming.—Obstruction of the articular disc between the condyle and articular eminence sufficient to interfere with translatory movement is called disc jamming. It can occur only if there is firm contact between condyle, disc, and eminence. It is not indicative of complete dislocation of the articular disc from the condyle. It can occur for different reasons. Excessive passive interarticular pressure, structural incompatibility between the sliding surfaces (for any reason, including functional remodeling), and damage sustained by the disc itself are frequent causes. It should be noted, however, that disc jamming may accompany (1) excessive biting force, (2) unusual, excessive, or strained jaw movements, or (3) momentary lack of muscular coordination. Movements and jaw positions can be learned that cause momentary disc jamming.[3] Learned, habitual "popping of the joints" is commonplace. Such disc jamming may occur without serious impairment of function or structural change in the disc-condyle complex, although such conditions no doubt predispose to damage. As long as disc-condyle complex function remains unimpaired, disc jamming usually occurs on a momentary basis. Such jamming may be demonstrated clinically by repeating the conditions of movement or position that induce it. When forced, such jamming may elicit momentary pain of disc-attachment type. Other movements and positions may remain symptom-free. Noise may be emitted when the obstruction is overcome. When the jamming relates specifically to power strokes, it may be decreased by biting against resistance on the symptomatic side. Occasionally, acute disc jamming may remain protracted, thus inducing acutely painful symptoms of discitis and eventually capsulitis.

Considerably more serious disc jamming may occur in conjunction with dysfunctional discal ligaments. This may complicate functional displacements of the articular disc (as subsequently discussed). Although such disc jamming may be momentary and may therefore simulate the acute condition described above (except that it is usually less painful and emits minimal noise when overcome), it may also induce protracted arrestment of the condylar movement. When this occurs, it is therapeutically expedient that it be differentiated from acute disc jamming. It also should be differentiated from blocked condylar movement due to a dislocated articular disc.

Protracted disc jamming associated with functional displacement of the articular disc may be identified by observing the following clinical criteria:

1. A protracted history of prior symptoms of functional displacement of the articular disc will be evident. This includes incidents of momentary (usually painless and relatively silent) disc jamming.

2. The condition remains relatively painless.

3. Movements within the range permitted are silent.

4. No acute malocclusion during maximum intercuspation is sensed.

5. Considerable protrusive and lateral movement may be permitted, due presumably to elongation of the discal ligaments.

6. When relieved by manipulation of the mandible, there is little or no noise or pain.

Blockage of Movement by a Dislocated Disc.—Blockage of the return phase of translatory movement by a dislocated and prolapsed articular disc as a result of *spontaneous* anterior dislocation is well known and generally understood. *Functional* dislocation, however, also occurs and is due to seriously impaired disc-condyle complex function. Reciprocal dislocation and reduction of such a dislocated articular disc occur during normal translatory cycles. Functional anterior dislocation of the disc results from contraction of the superior lateral pterygoid muscle; functional reduction results from posterior traction of the superior retrodiscal lamina. *Reduction, however, requires a full forward translatory movement.* If the dislocated disc blocks such movement, then the dislocation remains protracted. Such arrested mandibular movement is quite different from that of protracted disc jamming. In this situation, there no longer is surface contact of the condyle, disc, and articular eminence, and the disc is not wedged between the condyle and eminence. Rather, the disc is trapped anterior to the condyle *because of collapse of the articular disc space.* It is important therapeutically to differentiate protracted functional dislocation of the disc from protracted disc jamming as described above.

Protracted functional dislocation can be identified by observing the following clinical criteria:

1. A protracted history of serious disc interference, including reciprocal functional dislocation and reduction. This may include prior incidents of disc jamming also.

2. The condition becomes painful, with symptoms of acute retrodiscitis.

3. Movements of the mandible within the range permitted are noisy and grating.

4. Acute malocclusion during maximum intercuspation is sensed as ipsilateral overstressing of the posterior teeth.

5. Translatory movements of the condyle in protrusion and lateral excursion are restricted, proportionately with opening.

6. If manipulation of the mandible to relieve the blocking by the dislo-

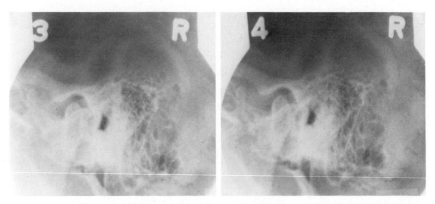

Fig 7–7.—Radiographs of right temporomandibular joint illustrate intracapsular restriction of mandibular movement. *Left,* lateral excursion to the opposite side. *Right,* maximum opening. Note that condylar movement in lateral excursion remains close to the closed position of the joint. The restriction in maximum opening is exactly the same. (Reproduced with permission from Bell W.E.: *Orofacial Pains: Differential Diagnosis,* ed. 2. Copyright © 1979 by Year Book Medical Publishers, Inc., Chicago.)

cated (usually distorted) articular disc is successful enough to permit a full forward movement of the condyle, automatic functional reduction occurs, usually painlessly and with little or no discal noise.

It should be noted that reduction of functional anterior dislocation of the articular disc is accomplished by traction of the fully stretched superior retrodiscal lamina. If such structure is not functional, then any anterior dislocation (functional, spontaneous, or traumatic) will be *permanent*.

Ankylosis.—Fibrous adhesions (or actual ossification) that unites the disc-condyle complex with the temporal articular facet limits condylar movement to the range permitted by the length of such adhesions. Rotatory movement is not affected. Such restriction of movement is silent and painless unless injured by abusive movements. The adhesions restrict condylar movement in protrusive and contralateral excursion. Radiographic confirmation is done by comparing the restricted condylar positions in open and lateral views with the closed-joint position. The location of the condyle in open and lateral positions nearly superimpose, and both remain fairly close to the closed position (Fig 7–7).

INTERFERENCE DURING MANDIBULAR MOVEMENT

Normally, movements of the disc-condyle complex along the articular eminence take place without any interference that would cause abnormal sensations, noises, movements, deviations of the midline incisal path, or pain (see chap. 5). Interference between the disc-condyle complex and the temporal articular surface presents clearly identifiable clinical evidence, namely:

· 1. Abnormal sensations that can be felt, such as rubbing, slipping, binding, or catching sensations.

2. Abnormal sounds that can be heard, such as clicking, popping, snapping, and grating noises.

3. Abnormal movements that can be seen, such as jerky or irregular movement or deviation of the midline incisal path.

4. Pain, if any, related temporally to the interference—either just prior to, with, or immediately following such interference.

Interference during mandibular movement is identified by various combinations of these symptoms as they relate to each other. *They should be considered together, not as isolated symptoms*. Good clinical evaluation of joint function requires that the interference responsible for such abnormal sensations, sounds, and movements be identified correctly. It is not enough just to recognize them; it is necessary to relate them to the functional abnormality that provokes them.

Although translatory cyclic movements of the disc-condyle complex are quite similar, whether they are for opening, protrusion, or lateral excursion, they are not necessarily identical. Likewise, symptoms of interference are not necessarily identical in the different jaw movements. Consideration should be given to interference behavior relative to lateral excursion to the opposite side. It is to be remembered that in lateral excursion, the balancing condyle follows a path of movement that is not straight forward, but moves medially. This movement is influenced by (1) the opposite joint (due to the effect of pivoting, restraint by the temporomandibular ligament, and sideways shift) and (2) the shape of the medial aspect of the articular eminence surface over which the translating disc-condyle complex moves. The difference between opening and lateral excursive movement, even in empty-mouth efforts, causes a difference in interference behavior also. These considerations should be kept in mind when comparing evidence of interference during the various movements of the mandible.

It should be noted that deviation of the midline incisal path during opening and closing is different from deflection, as described above. Deviation occurs as a neuromuscular habit pattern that develops in response to interference during mandibular movement. It may be considered a kind of compensatory mechanism for abnormality in the functioning of the disc-condyle complex. Deviation is discursive movement from the normal straight-line opening that returns again to the normal centered position.

Interference during mandibular movement should be considered according to how it relates to the translatory cycle, as follows:

1. That which occurs only in closed relationship of the joint (no part of the translatory cycle is involved).

2. That which occurs as the translatory cycle begins or ends.

3. That which occurs during the course and normal range of the translatory cycle.

4. That which occurs in the forward range of movement, beyond the limits of the normal translatory cycle, but short of dislocation.

5. That which occurs as spontaneous anterior dislocation during an overextended opening effort.

Interference That Occurs in Closed-Joint Position Only

ETIOLOGY.—Normally, maximum intercuspation of the teeth and resumption of a resting closed-joint position are wholly free of symptoms because the act of clenching the teeth should embody no strain on, or gross movement of, the articulating parts. It should consist only of a momentary increase in interarticular pressure as power is delivered by contraction of elevator muscles to bring the teeth into their fully occluded relationship.

But, if functional harmony is lacking between the muscle position of the joint (unclenched closed relationship) and the tooth form position (maximum intercuspation), the act of clenching the teeth causes movement between the disc-condyle complex and the articular eminence. As interarticular pressure increases due to elevator muscle action, such movement takes place under rapidly increasing friction, which tends to immobilize the articular disc against the eminence. Complications that develop depend on such factors as the inclination of the articular eminence, the force of the clenching effort, and the direction of movement so induced. As a result, frictional abuse may lead to deleterious change in the articular disc and the osseous-supported articular surfaces.

SYMPTOMS.—The clinical symptoms of interference of this type consist of:

1. A momentary sensation of stress or movement as the teeth are firmly clenched. This sensation is prevented by biting against a separator.

2. Discal noise, which may be heard as the teeth are brought into maximum intercuspation or immediately as biting force is released. This discal noise is prevented by biting against a separator.

3. Pain, if any, is a momentary disc-attachment arthralgic pain that occurs with maximum intercuspation. It is prevented by biting against a separator.

Radiographic confirmation is available if the occlusal disharmony is suf-

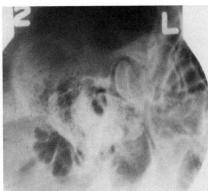

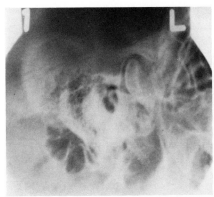

Left T-M Joint

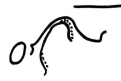

Fig 7–8.—Radiography confirms occlusal disharmony sufficient to displace condyle anteriorly when the teeth are occluded firmly. *Top,* radiographs of left temporomandibular joint in unclenched closed position *(left)* and clenched occluded position *(right)*. *Bottom,* tracings made from these films show condylar position in unclenched closed position as a *solid line,* in clenched occluded position as a *broken line.* Note that clenched occluded position is slightly anterior to the unclenched closed position. (Reproduced with permission from Bell W.E.: *Orofacial Pains: Differential Diagnosis,* ed. 2. Copyright © 1979 by Year Book Medical Publishers, Inc., Chicago.)

ficiently great to cause radiographically visible displacement of the condyle from unclenched to clenched occluded position and if such displacement takes place in the sagittal plane (Figs 7–8, 7–9).

Interference That Occurs as the Translatory Cycle Begins or Ends

ETIOLOGY.—Following maximum intercuspation, the elevator and superior lateral pterygoid muscles normally relax back to muscle tonus, thus permitting the joint to resume its resting closed position. When this takes place, the interarticular pressure returns to empty-mouth level, the articular disc space widens slightly, the superior lateral pterygoid muscle (by muscle tonus) rotates the articular disc anteriorly to properly fill the slightly widened disc space, and synovial fluid lubricates the joint surfaces. Thus, the joint is prepared for the next translatory cycle.

If, however, there is sufficient deterioration of the articular surfaces, this normal sequence may be interfered with. Maximum intercuspation may cause the articular disc to stick to the temporal surface. In that case, the

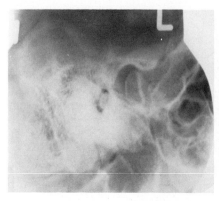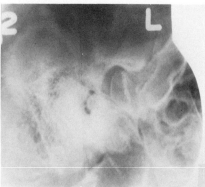

Left T-M Joint

Fig 7–9.—Radiography confirms occlusal disharmony sufficient to displace condyle posteriorly when the teeth are occluded firmly. *Top,* radiographs of left temporo-mandibular joint in unclenched closed position *(left)* and clenched occluded position *(right)*. *Bottom,* tracings made from these films show condylar position in un-clenched closed position as a *solid line,* in clenched occluded position as a *broken line.* Note that the clenched occluded position is slightly posterior to the unclenched closed position. (Reproduced with permission from Bell W.E.: *Oro-facial Pains: Differential Diagnosis,* ed. 2. Copyright © 1979 by Year Book Medical Publishers, Inc., Chicago.)

following translatory cycle cannot begin from the lubricated resting closed position. Instead, as the condyle moves forward, the discal collateral ligaments pull the disc free, thus emitting noise as it is suddenly replaced in position. Once this occurs, the disc-condyle complex completes a normal translatory cycle. If a power stroke ends in maximum intercuspation, the disc may tend to hang as the deteriorated articular surfaces drag against each other.

The chief cause of this type of interference is alteration in the articular surfaces at the closed-joint position. Several etiologic factors can cause such damage, namely

1. Trauma to the joint sustained when the teeth are in occlusion
2. Habitual hard biting force
3. Bruxism
4. Chronic occlusal disharmony

SYMPTOMS.—Such interference occurs after maximum intercuspation. Ordinarily, the symptoms take place as a new translatory movement is initiated following a biting stroke. They may also follow voluntary clenching of the teeth or bruxing. Or, they may consist of a single incidence of discal noise following a period of inactivity (e.g., first thing in the morning). Ordinarily, such symptoms do not occur if the translatory movement begins from the resting closed position. Such interference does not relate so much to protrusive or lateral excursions as to opening the mouth. Although the disc symptoms occur as the translatory cycle begins, the mouth may be opened several millimeters (up to 8 to 10 mm) before the noise is heard.

The interference that occurs as the translatory cycle ends relates to maximum intercuspation. If the cycle ends in a resting closed relationship instead of maximum intercuspation, the symptoms may not take place at all.

The severity of the deterioration in the articular surfaces in the closed position has considerable bearing on the symptoms produced. If such change is minor, it may require vigorous maximum intercuspation to induce interference. If damage is greater, less vigorous intercuspation of the teeth is required to initiate the symptoms.

The clinical symptoms of interference that occur just as the translatory cycle begins or ends are:

1. Following maximum intercuspation, voluntary clenching, or after a long period of inactivity, a sensation of tension or pulling may be felt as condylar movement begins. This is followed by a distinct click or pop. It may be associated with momentary pain. Following the initial symptoms, joint functioning appears to be normal.

2. As a power stroke ends in maximum intercuspation, the symptoms may be repeated, but in variable degree.

3. The symptoms are prevented by an occlusal stop that increases vertical dimension or slightly protrudes the mandible, which prevents the condyle from returning to the closed position.

Interference That Occurs During Normal Translatory Cycle

If there is structural compatibility between the moving parts and normal interarticular pressure, empty-mouth translatory cycles and power strokes are normally smooth and relatively silent. The inclination of the articular eminence bears importantly on joint function. Any discrepancy assumes greater significance in steeply inclined joints. This consideration has importance both diagnostically and therapeutically.

Interference that occurs during normal translatory cycles and power strokes stems from a variety of causes, some of minor significance, some constituting calamitous conditions of the joint. The causes may be grouped under three main headings, namely,

1. Excessive passive interarticular pressure
2. Structural incompatibility between the sliding parts
3. Impairment of disc-condyle complex function

The etiology and symptomatology of these groups will be considered separately.

EXCESSIVE PASSIVE INTERARTICULAR PRESSURE. —In spite of morphology and lack of precise structural harmony between the sliding parts, and, even in spite of some malfunctioning within the disc-condyle complex proper, cyclic movement of the mandible may remain free of interference, *providing the interarticular pressure is low*. If, however, there is relative increase in joint pressure, conditions that predispose to interference during sliding movements may be accentuated. Therefore, increased interarticular pressure may activate an otherwise nonsymptomatic condition into a clinical complaint.

If all conditions of the temporomandibular joint are normal, increased interarticular pressure alone does not induce interference with movement. The joints are constructed to function well under varying degrees of pressure. But, if some abnormality that predisposes to interference is present, increased interarticular pressure may become the *activating factor* that initiates symptoms.

Interarticular pressure is the product of muscle action (see chap. 4). It varies as elevator muscle action is brought to bear on resistance between the teeth in power strokes and maximum intercuspation.

The level of *passive* interarticular pressure, at the resting closed position of the joint and during empty-mouth translatory cycles, depends on *muscle tonus* of elevator masticatory muscles. Such tonus is not constant. It varies with emotional tension. During periods of increased emotional stress, the tonicity of elevator muscles increases, thus increasing the passive interarticular pressure within the joints. During such periods, interference may occur as symptoms of discal noise, sensations of interference, or even discomfort. Persons with conditions of this sort have a history of intermittent, recurring episodes of interference that relate to recurring periods of elevated emotional stress. A single emotional crisis can be sufficient to precipitate a symptomatic condition in the absence of a history of any prior occurrence.

Conditions that induce muscle splinting and myospasm activity also increase the passive interarticular pressure within the joints (see chaps. 4 and 6). Changes in the oral environment, sensed as injury or threat of injury, and increased oral consciousness may be answered by muscle splinting. Increased emotional tension may accentuate the problem. Thus, interarticular pressure may be increased sufficiently to activate symptoms of interference. Protracted muscle splinting may develop myospastic activity. Myospasm of elevator masticatory muscles, regardless of cause, predisposes to such interference.

It should be noted that, if interference is great enough to actually obstruct the articular disc and thereby arrest mandibular movement, it is classified as *restriction of mandibular movement*.

The clinical indications that interference may be due to excessive passive interarticular pressure are:

1. Occurrence of symptoms with or following increased emotional stress or crisis.

2. Sudden onset of symptoms that accompany an acute muscle disorder of the masticatory apparatus.

3. Variability, recurrence, or periodicity in symptom behavior.

Structural incompatibility between sliding surfaces.—Lack of structural harmony between the upper surface of the disc-condyle complex and the articular eminence predisposes to interference. Regardless of the particular type of disharmony or its cause, the symptoms are (1) sensations of hanging or catching, (2) noises such as clicking or popping, and (3) irregular or arrested movement. Deviation of the midline incisal path with opening and closing is commonplace. Sometimes, discomfort also accompanies the interference. All such symptoms relate to each other in that they tend to occur each time similar movements are made. They persist and may become slowly worse with time.

The chronic nature of interference of this kind appears to favor the development of habit patterns of opening and closing that compensate for the interference in the form of deviation of the incisal path. It should be noted, however, that if movements are speeded up, the interference may become more evident. Interference due to structural incompatibility relates not only to the force and speed of movements, but also to the interarticular pressure within the joint.

Some structural incompatibility relates to the inclination of the articular eminence. As has been discussed previously (chap. 5), the steeper the articular eminence, the greater the functional burden placed on the disc-condyle complex to execute translatory cycles smoothly and silently. Extremely steep joints may show evidence of minor interference, especially when movements are rapid or forceful.

Some structural interference may occur as the result of a developmental anomaly, such as a gross malformation, lack of harmony in the size or shape of the sliding parts as they relate to each other and to the opposite joint, and remodeling and aberrations of growth from any cause. Some structural interference is acquired as the result of trauma. A fairly frequent cause of interference has to do with minor trauma sustained when the jaws are separated, thus causing the damage to occur along the incline of the articular eminence. Interference is noticed when the disc-condyle complex slides over the site of damage during translatory cycles. More severe trauma may lead to hypertrophic growth and other deformation at the site of injury. Some sequelae of trauma are sufficiently great to be visible radiographically.

Structural interference may occur as the result of deleterious change in response to such things as habitual abusive use, mannerisms, and unusual functional conditions imposed on the masticatory apparatus. Most such etiologic factors are obvious, e.g., habitually biting on a pipestem, cigar, pencil, or other object held between the teeth; chewing on fingernails, tooth picks, rubber bands, or bubble gum; and mannerisms involving protrusive or lateral movements due to nervousness, oral consciousness, or dental appliances. Chronic occlusal interference during lateral excursions that cause abnormal movements in the balancing joint may cause some deterioration. Another cause is restricted translatory movement in the opposite joint. When normal movement is restrained, the act of opening and closing causes the unrestrained condyle to move medially. Such unnatural movement tends to induce deleterious changes in the translating joint, thus leading to functional interference. Another cause of structural disharmony between the sliding articular surfaces is change in the subarticular osseous structure due to degenerative or rheumatoid arthritis.

It should be noted that when the interference is due to structural incompatibility of the sliding surfaces, any increase in the articular disc space decreases the symptoms. This takes place on the biting side during power strokes. *Therefore, patients with this complaint may find themselves doing their hard chewing on the symptomatic side.*

The clinical indications that interference is due to structural incompatibility between the sliding surfaces are:

1. Discrete, precise, and unchanging symptoms that occur with little or no variation as similar movements are executed.

2. Deviations of the incisal path that minimize the interference. More rapid movements may make the symptoms more evident.

3. Chronicity, persistence, or resistance to therapy.

4. Decrease in interference by chewing on the symptomatic side.

5. Chronic occlusal disharmony that alters movements in the balancing joint.

6. Restricted movement in the opposite joint.

IMPAIRED DISC-CONDYLE COMPLEX FUNCTION.—Considerably more serious causes of interference have to do with conditions that disrupt normal functioning of the disc-condyle complex. These include (1) arrested hinge movement between the articular disc and condyle, (2) damaged articular

disc, (3) dysfunctional discal ligaments, and (4) dysfunctional superior retrodiscal lamina.

Adhesions Between the Articular Disc and Condyle.—Adhesions may
unite the mandibular condyle and articular disc, thus preventing normal
rotatory movements that are essential to the functioning of the temporomandibular joint. This can occur as the result of trauma, infection, and
rheumatoid arthritis. It is a rare condition. When rotatory movement does
not occur, translation of the condyle cannot incorporate smooth gliding action that results from surface-to-surface contact of articular disc with the
articular eminence. Rather, the immobilized disc remains in a fixed relationship with the condyle, thus skidding forward with only a portion of the
disc in contact with the temporal articular surface. This constitutes *partial
dislocation* or subluxation. The whole translatory cycle consists of an irregular, noisy, skidding movement forward and backward.

The clinical indication of this condition is the presence of symptoms similar to those of joint hypermobility, except that they occur throughout the
entire translatory cycle rather than with extended opening only.

Damaged Articular Disc.—Damage to the articular disc may consist of
roughening, thinning, perforation, or fracture. Roughening of the disc
causes a grating interference throughout the translatory cycle, punctuated
at times by more discrete symptoms at points of greater interference. Thinning does very little to increase symptoms unless it involves the anterior
or posterior areas disproportionately. If thinning occurs in conjunction with
elongation of discal ligaments, then thinning anteriorly predisposes to functional displacement of the disc posteriorly during full forward translatory
cycles, whereas thinning posteriorly predisposes to anterior functional displacement during power strokes. Perforations of the disc may alter joint
function through disruption of normal hydrodynamics of synovial fluid,
about which little is presently known. Fracture of the disc adds little to the
symptoms unless the fractured parts are separated or override each other.
Both conditions cause acute malocclusion of the ipsilateral posterior teeth,
sensed during maximum intercuspation. Separated fragments cause a sensation of overstressed posterior teeth; overriding fragments cause disocclusion of the posterior teeth.

Deleterious change in the articular disc occurs as the result of microtraumas from abusive use, structural interference during jaw movements, frictional displacement during maximum intercuspation, and overloading. The
most important predisposing factor is chronic occlusal disharmony, and paramount among exciting causes are bruxism and habitual hard chewing.
Acute trauma occasionally is a factor. It should be noted that damaged

articular discs and dysfunctional discal ligaments are facets of a common problem of functional abuse.

The clinical indications suggestive of a damaged articular disc are:

1. Continuous grating noise throughout the translatory cycle, punctuated by discrete symptoms at points of greater interference.

2. Functional displacements of the disc during power strokes and/or full forward translatory movements.

3. Acute malocclusion sensed as overstressed or disoccluded ipsilateral posterior teeth during maximum intercuspation.

Dysfunctional Discal Ligaments.—The collateral ligaments that attach the articular disc to the medial and lateral poles of the mandibular condyle convert the disc-condyle complex into a simple hinge joint. They permit freedom of rotatory movement in the anteroposterior direction but *resist stresses that tend to displace the disc from the condyle in any direction*. These structures cause the disc to follow the condyle wherever it goes. Their presence is essential to normal functioning of the temporomandibular joint.

All stresses that tend to displace the disc from the condyle are brought to bear on the discal ligaments. This includes the conditions that cause deleterious changes in the disc proper, namely, abusive use, structural interference during jaw movements, frictional displacement during maximum intercuspation, and overloading. Occlusal disharmony, accentuated especially by habitual hard chewing and bruxism, is the chief condition responsible for deleterious changes in the ligaments. Acute trauma sometimes may be a factor.

Resultant damage to the discal ligaments may consist of elongation, structural change that renders them less effective as ligamentous structures, or actual detachment from the condyle. Although such change almost invariably affects both ligaments to some degree, the extent may be disproportionate between the two. All such damage seriously disrupts functioning and is irreversible.

It should be noted that these ligaments, like all true ligaments, are composed of nonelastic collagenous tissue. Under stress, they do not stretch. When stress is excessive over a period of time, they may lengthen *permanently*. Such elongation permits unnatural movement between the disc and condyle, the amount depending on the extent of elongation. This kind of damage is commonplace and usually is accompanied by destructive change in the articular disc as well.

Dysfunctional discal ligaments convert the joint from a ginglymo-arthrodial (hinge-sliding) joint into an arthrodial-arthrodial (sliding-sliding) joint. The disc may then be displaced posteriorly by traction of the superior retrodiscal lamina during forward phases of the translatory cycle. It may be displaced anteriorly by contraction of the superior lateral pterygoid muscle during power strokes and maximum intercuspation. As a result, smooth, silent, gliding movement during translatory cycles is lost. Movements may become irregular and noisy. More discrete symptoms may occur at points of greater interference.

Two clinical symptom displays may develop as the result of dysfunctional discal ligaments in conjunction with damaging change in the articular disc, namely, functional displacement and functional dislocation of the articular disc. These conditions should be identified and differentiated.

The deleterious change that leads to these conditions has to do with thinning of the articular disc in the normally thicker anterior or posterior portions, so that precise confinement of the disc as determined by the width of the articular disc space is jeopardized. As long as adequate contour of the disc remains, gross displacement is not likely to occur, even though translatory movements may be noisy and irregular due to sliding between the articular disc and condyle. When thinning of the anterior or posterior portion of the disc is sufficient, some displacement is permitted, depending on the forces applied by the superior lateral pterygoid muscle and the superior retrodiscal lamina. The amount of such displacement depends on the extent of elongation of the discal collateral ligaments as well as deterioration of the disc itself.

Functional Displacement of the Disc.—If the deleterious change in the articular disc involves the posterior portion and if the discal ligaments are elongated, the disc in the occluded relationship of the joint remains displaced anteriorly due to contraction of the superior lateral pterygoid muscle. As opening begins, the condyle moves forward on the displaced disc until it is seated against its thicker anterior portion, by which it is then moved. Minor noise may be elicited or the interference sensed subjectively. The disc remains seated on the condyle throughout an empty-mouth cycle until again displaced by contraction of the superior lateral pterygoid muscle. This may occur suddenly if the return movement is rapid or powered, the contraction of the superior lateral pterygoid muscle forcefully displacing the disc anteriorly, thus emitting discal noise. The disc remains anteriorly displaced through maximum intercuspation and the resting closed position. Then the sequence begins again. Momentary or protracted disc jamming (locking) may take place as previously described.

If the deleterious change in the articular disc involves the anterior portion and the disc ligaments are elongated, then, when the condyle begins to move forward (especially following maximum intercuspation), the disc may remain against the fossa articular surface until tugged free by the elongated discal ligaments and brought back into position on the condyle by the extended (but not contracted) superior lateral pterygoid muscle. This may initiate a distinct click, the point of opening at which it occurs being determined largely by the extent of elongation of the discal ligaments. With continued opening the disc is again displaced posteriorly by the extended superior retrodiscal lamina. Discal noise may or may not occur, depending on the rapidity of movement. If the return movement is empty-mouth and slow (nonpowered), the disc may remain in posterior displacement until replaced by muscle tonus action of the superior lateral pterygoid muscle in the closed-joint relationship. If the return movement is rapid or powered, however, the contraction of the superior lateral pterygoid muscle forcefully replaces the displaced disc on the condyle, emitting discrete discal noise. Maximum intercuspation sets the stage for repetition of the sequence. To demonstrate this symptom display clinically, it may be necessary to initiate the preparation for the first click by firmly clenching the teeth and then produce the second by a rapid or forceful closure. Momentary or protracted disc jamming (locking) may take place also.

It should be noted that in such functional displacements, the articular disc undergoes only partial dislocation. The disc may slide bodily on the condyle, but it remains between the condylar and temporal articular surfaces, *thus preventing collapse of the articular disc space*. Although momentary or protracted arrested mandibular movement may occur due to disc jamming, blockage of condylar movement by a dislocated disc does not take place.

Symptoms of such interference are usually *increased* by chewing on the symptomatic side, a point that may help differentiate this kind of complaint from interference due to excessive passive interarticular pressure or incompatible articular surfaces.

Functional Dislocation of the Articular Disc.—Functional dislocation of the articular disc is possible when the border of the disc is thinned enough to permit it to be *pulled through* the articular disc space and when the discal ligaments are sufficiently nonfunctional to permit such gross displacement of the disc to take place.

If the posterior border of the disc is thinned sufficiently, functional dislocation in an *anterior* direction can occur during power strokes and maximum intercuspation. This is especially true on the biting side, as the articular disc space normally widens due to biting against resistance. The force that dislocates the disc is the strong contraction of the superior lateral pterygoid muscle in conjunction with the execution of power strokes and maximum intercuspation. With anterior dislocation, the articular disc space collapses and the disc remains in front of the condyle until functional reduction is accomplished by posterior traction of the superior retrodiscal lamina during a full forward translatory cycle. Thus, true reciprocal symptoms occur: first, with the dislocation during a biting effort, followed by reduction symptoms during a forward translatory cycle. If the first does not occur, neither does the second. It should be noted that since functional reduction requires a full forward translatory cyclic movement, such reduction is impossible if the dislocated disc blocks such movement. In that case, the disc remains in front of the condyle. Symptoms of such protracted dislocation consist of blocked translatory movement, grating sounds during the movements that do occur, acute malocclusion sensed as overstressed ipsilateral posterior teeth during maximum intercuspation, and increasing retrodiscitis.

If the anterior border of the articular disc is thinned sufficiently, functional dislocation *in a posterior direction* can occur during a full forward translatory cycle. At that time, posterior force is applied by the fully stretched elastic superior retrodiscal lamina. The dislocated disc will remain behind the condyle until functional reduction is accomplished by anterior traction exerted by the superior lateral pterygoid muscle during a power stroke or closing effort. Reciprocal symptoms occur, first with the dislocation during a forward translatory movement, followed by reduction during the return movement. *Protracted posterior dislocation does not take place.*

The clinical indications suggestive of dysfunctional discal ligaments are:

1. More or less continuous irregular movements and grating type noise throughout the translatory cycle, punctuated by discrete symptoms at points of greater interference.

2. Symptoms of reciprocal functional displacement. Usually such symptoms are accentuated following maximum intercuspation and by rapid closure or power strokes. Chewing on the symptomatic side usually accentuates the symptoms.

3. Symptoms of reciprocal functional dislocation and reduction of the articular disc, related to power strokes and full forward translatory movements.

4. Blocked translatory movement associated with acute malocclusion sensed as overstressed ipsilateral posterior teeth during maximum intercuspation.

Dysfunctional Superior Retrodiscal Lamina.—The superior retrodiscal lamina is the only joint structure that exerts traction on the articular disc in a posterior direction. This takes place only during the forward phase of a translatory cycle. The function of the superior retrodiscal lamina is to rotate the disc posteriorly and, thus, reduce the danger of spontaneous anterior dislocation at the critical forward position just prior to the return phase of the cycle.

Because of its favorable location, the superior lamina is well protected from condylar encroachment and, therefore, is seldom damaged even by traumatic force. This is fortunate indeed because normal disc action is lost during the forward phase of translatory cycles if the lamina becomes dysfunctional. Not only may symptoms of discal interference become evident, but also the danger of spontaneous anterior dislocation is increased.

Traumatic severance of the superior retrodiscal lamina from the articular disc renders any prolapse or anterior dislocation of the disc *permanent* because no other structure within the joint can be manipulated in such a way as to replace the disc on the condyle.[4]

The clinical indications suggestive of a dysfunctional superior retrodiscal lamina are:

1. History of prior trauma to the mandible.

2. Irregular noisy movements, especially in the forward phase of translatory cycles prior to power strokes.

3. Protracted *spontaneous* anterior dislocation that cannot be reduced.

4. Protracted *functional* anterior dislocation of the articular disc that cannot be reduced.

Interference That Occurs Anterior to Normal Translation

Smooth, relatively silent, sliding movement in the temporomandibular joint depends on normal rotation of the articular disc on the condyle to maintain surface-to-surface contact between the sliding parts. Wide opening entails posterior rotation of the disc. When the combined rotatory movement from opening and translation reaches the limit imposed by the posterior border of the condylar articular facet, further rotatory movement is arrested. Then, extended opening of the mouth exceeds normal translatory movement. When mouth-opening is beyond normal, it takes place without benefit of continuous surface contact of the sliding parts. The disc-condyle complex skids along the anterior slope of the articular eminence with only its posterior border in contact (see Fig 3–7). This partial dislocation induces clinical symptoms consisting of an initial pause, then a sudden jumping forward of the condyle, accompanied by noise and sometimes discomfort. This condition is referred to as subluxation or joint hypermobility.

The etiology of such interference is habitual overextension of opening beyond normal limits. It does not usually occur with protrusive or lateral movements. It is more likely to occur with very steep joints. Subluxation predisposes to spontaneous anterior dislocation.

SYMPTOMS.—The clinical symptoms of interference of this kind include the following:

1. As the mouth is opened fully, a momentary pause is followed by the condyle suddenly leaping forward to its full anterior limit.

2. This jerky movement of the condyle is accompanied by noise and sometimes minor discomfort.

3. These symptoms do not take place with protrusive or lateral excursive movements unless the mouth is opened also.

Interference Caused by Spontaneous Anterior Dislocation

When the mouth is opened widely, the disc-condyle complex is situated at the full forward position of the translatory cycle with the disc rotated posteriorly by the stretched superior retrodiscal lamina. At this critical moment when forward condylar movement is arrested by the taut posterior capsular ligament, further effort to open the mouth or any *premature* contraction of the superior lateral pterygoid muscle may result in spontaneous anterior dislocation of the joint (see Fig 8–1).

SYMPTOMS.—The clinical symptoms of spontaneous anterior dislocation are:

1. Inability to close the mouth after an overextended opening. As the posterior teeth (or edentulous ridges) come into contact, the anteriors remain widely apart.

2. Discomfort, if any, is due to the application of force in an attempt to close the mouth.

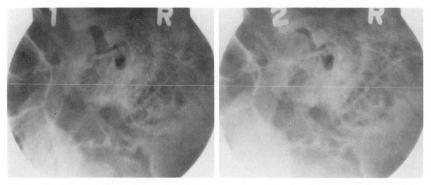

Fig 7–10.—Radiographs of right temporomandibular joint illustrate muscle-induced acute malocclusion caused by myospastic activity in the right lateral pterygoid muscle. *Left,* unclenched closed position; *right,* clenched occluded position. Note that the unclenched closed position is anteriorly displaced by contraction of the right lateral pterygoid muscle. Maximum intercuspation forces condyle posteriorly into its usual occluded relationship.

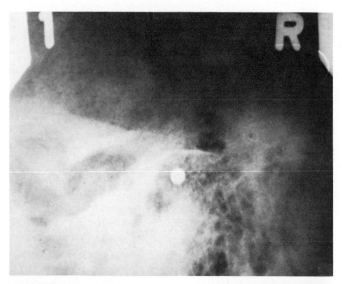

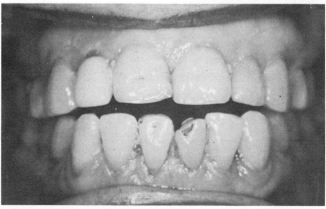

Fig 7–11.—Illustration of joint-induced acute malocclusion caused by rapid resorption of condylar osseous structure from rheumatoid arthritis. *Top,* radiograph of temporomandibular joint showing bizarre osseous resorption that reduces vertical height of mandibular ramus. (Reproduced with permission from Bell W.E.: *Orofacial Pains: Differential Diagnosis,* ed. 2. Copyright © 1979 by Year Book Medical Publishers, Inc., Chicago.) *Bottom,* photograph of resulting progressive anterior open-bite. (From Bell W.E.: Management of temporomandibular problems, in Goldman H.M., Gilmore H.W., Royer R.Q., et al. (eds.): *Current Therapy In Dentistry.* St. Louis, C.V. Mosby Co., 1970, vol. 4. Reproduced with permission.)

ACUTE MALOCCLUSION

Another symptom of masticatory dysfunction is acute malocclusion—that which occurs suddenly in conjunction with other evidence of dysfunction and about which the subject is fully aware. Such malocclusion is sensed subjectively as a change in the way the teeth occlude. It usually is accompanied by some discomfort when the teeth are brought forcefully into maximum intercuspation. Such discomfort usually is reduced by biting against a separator that prevents bringing the teeth into their fully occluded relationship.

Acute malocclusion may be induced by (1) muscle action or (2) sudden change in the relationship of the disc-condyle complex to the articular eminence.

Muscle-Induced Acute Malocclusion

Most muscle-induced malocclusion results from spasm of the lateral pterygoid muscle. The condyle is drawn forward on the affected side, thus causing disocclusion of the posterior teeth and premature contact of the anteriors contralaterally. This condition can be confirmed radiographically by comparing the unclenched closed position with the clenched

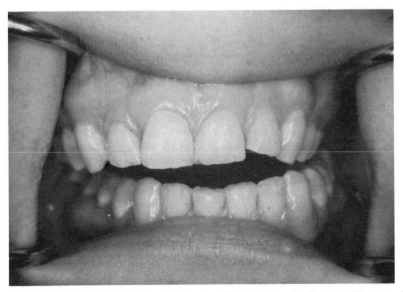

Fig 7–12.—Acute malocclusion due to rheumatoid arthritis in a 24-year-old woman. Anterior open-bite was rapidly progressive.

position. The condyle is displaced anteriorly in the resting closed position (Fig 7–10).

Myospasm involving elevator muscles may induce acute malocclusion of a less dramatic type. Such may be evident only subjectively. Spasm of the masseter muscle tends to displace the mandible laterally; spasm of the medial pterygoid displaces it medially.

Joint-Induced Acute Malocclusion

Sudden change in the relationship of the disc-condyle complex with the articular eminence causes acute malocclusion. This may occur as the result of gross trauma to, or rapid deterioration of, the osseous surfaces (Figs 7–11 and 7–12), overriding or separation of the parts of a fractured articular disc, dislocation of the disc from the condyle, swelling of the retrodiscal tissue, or accumulation of excessive fluid within the joint cavity from inflammatory effusion or hemarthrosis (Fig 7–13). It may occur iatrogenically as a result of local anesthesia of the joint or the injection of a solution into the joint cavity.

Symptoms of Acute Malocclusion

The clinical indications suggestive of acute (symptomatic) malocclusion that may be a symptom of masticatory dysfunction are:

1. Recent obvious change in the occlusion of which the patient is aware and about which he complains.

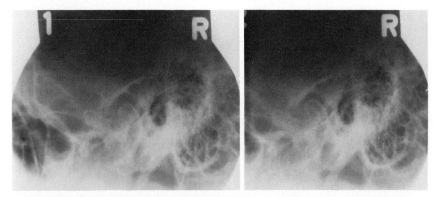

Fig 7–13.—Radiographs of right temporomandibular joint illustrate joint-induced acute malocclusion caused by inflammatory effusion of fluid within the joint cavity. *Left,* unclenched closed position; *Right,* clenched occluded position. Note that unclenched closed position is inferiorly displaced by the presence of excessive intracapsular fluid. Maximum intercuspation forces the condyle superiorly into the usual occluded relationship.

2. Such altered occlusion occurs in conjunction with other evidence of masticatory dysfunction or pain.

3. Accompanying pain is increased with maximum intercuspation and decreased by biting against a separator ipsilaterally.

REFERENCES

1. Bell W.E.: Temporomandibular joint, in Goldman H.M., Forrest S.P., Byrd D.L., et al. (eds.): *Current Therapy in Dentistry*. St. Louis, C.V. Mosby Co., 1968, vol. 3, pp. 557–584.
2. Farrar W.B.: Diagnosis and treatment of anterior dislocation of the articular disc. *N.Y. J. Dent*. 41:348, 1971.
3. Krogh-Poulsen W.G.: Discussion, in Blaschke D.D.: Arthrography of the temporomandibular joint, in Solberg W.K., Clark G.T. (eds.): *Temporomandibular Joint Problems*. Chicago, Quintessence Publishing Co., 1980, pp. 69–91.
4. Shira R.B., Alling C.C.: Traumatic injuries involving the temporomandibular joint articulation, in Schwartz L.L., Chayes C.M. (eds.): *Facial Pain and Mandibular Dysfunction*. Philadelphia, W.B. Saunders Co., 1968, pp. 129–139.

8 / Categories of Temporomandibular Disorders

ONE CAN RECOGNIZE only what one is familiar with. Identification of a particular condition requires the examiner to be conversant with the possible disorders he may encounter. The final step in programming the examiner's CNS computer, therefore, is to establish a good understanding of the various categories of disorders that afflict the masticatory apparatus. It is not enough to merely establish that a problem of the temporomandibular joint exists.

Disorders of the masticatory apparatus have similarities and differences. It is by their similarities that they can be grouped into various classes of conditions. It is by their differences that individual disorders within each group can be identified. Establishing an accurate clinical diagnosis demands knowledge of the similarities and differences of various masticatory disorders. One cannot hope to recognize a condition that he does not know exists, nor can he identify it accurately if he does not know how it compares with other disorders of the system.

The ultimate objective of diagnosis should be to name correctly the disorder, establish its location, understand its probable etiology, and predict with reasonable certainty its future course. Once this is accomplished, therapeutic management of the condition should be predictively effective.

CLASSIFICATION OF TEMPOROMANDIBULAR DISORDERS

Depending on their clinical similarities, temporomandibular disorders may be grouped into the five main classes listed in Table 8–1. In order to identify different disorders within each particular class, certain clinical features should be considered. They will be listed in the following sequence:

1. Features in the history that are etiologically significant
2. Symptoms of masticatory pain
3. Symptoms of restriction of mandibular movement
4. Symptoms of interference during mandibular movement
5. Symptoms of acute malocclusion
6. Radiographic confirmation (if needed)

Each group of temporomandibular disorders has certain features in common (Table 8–2).

Acute muscle disorders are characterized by sudden onset, changeable-

TABLE 8–1.—CLASSIFICATION OF TEMPOROMANDIBULAR DISORDERS

ACUTE MUSCLE DISORDERS
  Masticatory muscle splinting
  Masticatory muscle spasm (MPD syndrome)
    Elevator muscle spasm
    Lateral pterygoid muscle spasm
    Elevator and lateral pterygoid spasm
  Masticatory muscle inflammation (myositis)

DISC-INTERFERENCE DISORDERS OF THE JOINT
  Class I interference (at closed-joint position)
  Class II interference (as translatory cycle begins)
  Class III interference (during normal cycle)
    Excessive passive interarticular pressure
    Structural incompatibility
    Impaired disc-condyle complex
      Adhesions between disc and condyle
      Damaged articular disc
      Dysfunctional discal ligaments
        Functional displacement of disc
        Functional dislocation of disc
      Dysfunctional superior retrodiscal lamina
  Class IV interference (partial dislocation anterior to cycle)
  Spontaneous anterior dislocation

INFLAMMATORY DISORDERS OF THE JOINT
  Synovitis and capsulitis
  Retrodiscitis
  Inflammatory arthritis
    Traumatic arthritis
    Degenerative arthritis
    Infectious arthritis
    Rheumatoid arthritis
    Hyperuricemia

CHRONIC MANDIBULAR HYPOMOBILITIES
  Contracture of elevator muscle
    Myostatic contracture
    Myofibrotic contracture
  Capsular fibrosis
  Ankylosis
    Fibrous ankylosis
    Osseous ankylosis

GROWTH DISORDERS OF THE JOINT
  Aberration of development
  Acquired change in structure
  Neoplasia

ness, and recurrence. *Pain of myogenous type dominates the symptom complex.* Such pain relates intimately to muscle action—contracting and stretching. The pain is more or less continuous but may be quite variable. Secondary central excitatory effects, such as referred pains and secondary muscle spasms, may complicate the symptom picture. Usually, some re-

TABLE 8–2.—IDENTIFYING FEATURES OF CATEGORIES OF TEMPOROMANDIBULAR DISORDERS

	ACUTE MUSCLE DISORDERS	DISC-INTERFERENCE DISORDERS	INFLAMMATORY DISORDERS	CHRONIC MANDIBULAR HYPOMOBILITIES	GROWTH DISORDERS
History	Sudden onset Changeable Recurrent	Insidious onset Persistent Progressive	Prior trauma, noninflammatory joint disorder, illness	Prior trauma or infection Protracted course	Insidious structural change precedes symptoms
Masticatory pain	Dominates complaint Myalgia relates to muscle action Continuous but variable; may see secondary effects	If any, arthralgia of disc attachment type; intermittent	Dominates complaint Arthralgia of inflammatory type relates to joint function Continuous but variable; may see secondary effects	None, unless subjected to abusive movement	If any, due to progressive structural dysfunction
Restriction of movement	If any, extracapsular, due to shortened, rigid, or swollen elevator muscle	If any, intracapsular, due to jamming or dislocation of disc	If any, due to capsulitis, disc jamming, preexistent arthropathy, extra-articular disease or secondary spasm	Dominates complaint Due to ankylosis, capsular fibrosis, or contracture of elevator muscle	If any, due to progressive structural dysfunction
Interference during movement	If any, due to increased interarticular pressure or lateral pterygoid spasm	Dominates complaint Abnormal sensations, noises, and movements due to disc interference	If any, due to disruption of disc-condyle complex function	None	None, unless due to disruption of disc-condyle complex function

Acute malocclusion	If any, due chiefly to lateral pterygoid spasm	If any, due to fracture or dislocation of disc	If any, due to intracapsular fluid, retrodiscal swelling, or bone loss	None	If any, due to rapid osseous change
Radiographic confirmation	May be positive for restricted movement or gross malocclusion	May be positive for malocclusion or structural change in disc	May be positive for restricted movement or change in bone or disc space	Positive for location of restricted movement	Positive for structural aberration

striction of mandibular movement is evident. Such restriction is identified as extracapsular in type. It results from spastic or inflamed elevator muscles. If any interference during mandibular movement is clinically evident, it results from increased interarticular pressure due to elevator muscle spasm. Acute malocclusion is due chiefly to lateral pterygoid myospasm and only slightly to elevator muscle shortening. Radiography may confirm extracapsular restriction of movement or gross malocclusion.

Disc-interference disorders of the joint are characterized by insidious onset, persistence, and progressiveness. Masticatory pain may not be a prominent feature. When present, it is arthralgic and of the disc-attachment variety, clearly intermittent, and not prone to induce secondary central excitatory effects. Restriction of mandibular movement, if present, is due to jamming of, or blockage by, a damaged articular disc. *The dominant feature of disc-interference disorders is interference during mandibular movement*, manifested by abnormal sensations, noises, and movements. These symptoms include (1) sensations of binding, rubbing, or catching, (2) noises such as clicking, popping, snapping, or grating, and (3) irregular, rough, jerky movements or deviations of the midline incisal path during mouth opening. Such interference may cause jamming of the articular disc or functional dislocation. Acute malocclusion, if any, results from fracture or dislocation of the articular disc. Radiographic confirmation may be positive for gross malocclusion and structural change in the articular disc space or the subarticular bone.

Inflammatory disorders of the joint are preceded by trauma, noninflammatory disc-interference disorder, or a contributing illness, such as rheumatoid disease, hyperuricemia, or infection. *The dominant feature is arthralgic pain of inflammatory type* that relates intimately to joint function. Although quite variable, it is more or less continuous and, therefore, may excite secondary centrally induced effects, such as referred pains and muscle spasm activity, which confuse the symptom picture. Restriction of movement may or may not be evident. Unless such restriction results from the disorder that precedes the inflammatory condition, it is due to capsular inflammation or disruption of disc-condyle complex functioning. Secondary myospasm or other extra-articular condition may impose a measure of extracapsular restriction of mandibular movement also. Interference during mandibular movement, if any, is due to disc-condyle complex dysfunction. Acute malocclusion may result from accumulation of intracapsular fluid, swelling of the retrodiscal tissue, or very rapid resorption of subarticular bone. Radiography may confirm the location of restricted mandibular movement or significant change in the articular disc space or subarticular bone structure.

Chronic mandibular hypomobilities have a protracted course, preceded as they are by trauma or infection that may date back many years, even to infancy or childbirth. These conditions are chronic and painless unless aggravated by abusive use or excessive movement. Such aggravation may induce inflammation, thus causing the complaint to be classified initially as an inflammatory disorder of the joint. *The dominant feature is restriction of mandibular movement.* Extracapsular restriction results from contracture of an elevator muscle, capsular restriction from capsular fibrosis, and intracapsular restriction from ankylosis. These conditions are not associated with symptoms of interference during mandibular movement or acute malocclusion. Radiographic confirmation is positive for location of the cause of restricted movement and is essential to accurate diagnosis.

Growth disorders of the joint are characterized by insidious structural change that precedes clinical symptoms of masticatory pain or dysfunction. If masticatory pain or alteration of mandibular movement occurs, it is due to progressive dysfunction imposed by the growth aberration. No interference during mandibular movement is present unless or until the growth problem causes disruption of normal disc-condyle complex functioning. Acute malocclusion, if any, results from rapid osseous change. Radiographic confirmation is positive for identifying the structural aberration present and is essential to accurate diagnosis.

Although interference disorders, chronic mandibular hypomobilities, and growth disorders have clinical features that clearly identify them individually, acute muscle disorders and inflammatory conditions of the joint may have clinical symptoms that are much alike and therefore may be confused diagnostically. Accurate identification, however, is necessary, because the treatment for these two conditions is not the same.

ROLE OF EMOTIONAL TENSION

Sustained emotional tension plays an important role etiologically in many temporomandibular disorders.[4, 6] Such tension has to do with stressful life situations and results from the burden of being human. The masseter is among the first of the skeletal muscles to undergo protracted contraction as a result of stressful life situations.[11]

The presence of emotional tension should not imply that a serious psychological problem exists. All persons are subject to emotional stress. The signs of elevated emotional tension may develop suddenly. Usually, however, a less obvious, slow, smoldering buildup of tension accumulates from a variety of stressful situations, with no one incident being particularly decisive. Consequently, the emotional level rises and falls in a rhythmic pattern. Then some situation arises that adds just enough to an already high level of emotional tension that a crisis ensues. It may appear that such particular experience is responsible for the crisis, when actually it may have been no more than the straw that broke the camel's back. Learning to understand and successfully cope with life's stresses is a major challenge to modern man.

Emotional stress increases muscle tonus, thus altering the passive interarticular pressure in joints. In the craniomandibular articulation, such interarticular pressure increases the task of the disc-condyle complex to maintain continuous sharp contact of the articulating surfaces during all jaw movements and masticatory forces. Emotional stress is important in bruxism, not only in inducing it, but making it more destructive, as well. Emotional stress may be an essential activating factor in otherwise dormant and nonsymptomatic temporomandibular conditions. It is important both diagnostically and therapeutically, therefore, that emotional stress be recognized and evaluated.

Two important criteria serve to identify the presence of unusually high emotional stress. They may be framed in the form of questions to the subject:

1. Do you show ill temper and impatience with people and situations, especially trivialities, without justifiable provocation? Do you overreact to insignificant annoyances? Are you very easily offended? Do people make you nervous by their mere presence?

2. Do you go to bed more tired than your daily activities justify? And wake up the same way?

ACUTE MUSCLE DISORDERS

Each of the main categories of temporomandibular disorders consists of different conditions associated with typical, identifiable clinical features. Some such groups are comprised of subgroups (see Table 8–1). It is important that the particular complaint be recognized and identified as accurately as possible because effective therapy depends on it. Many clinical complaints consist of more than a single temporomandibular disorder that should be recognized, and some represent transitional phases from one condition to another.

No doubt, acute disorders involving the masticatory muscles are most frequent. Acute muscle disorders have certain features in common:

1. Myogenous type pain is a prominent feature of all *acute* muscle disorders. Such pain is elicited or aggravated by manual palpation or functional manipulation. It relates intimately to masticatory function.

2. They present some measure of extracapsular restriction of mandibular movement, induced by the inhibitory influence of pain, if not by structural muscle change.

3. Some degree of muscle-induced acute malocclusion is frequently present.

The acute myogenous complaints may be classified clinically as muscle splinting, muscle spasm, and muscle inflammation (Table 8–3). Various transition phases may occur between these disorders.

Masticatory Muscle Splinting

Muscle splinting is regarded *clinically* as a CNS-induced hypertonicity of a muscle(s) that occurs in response to altered proprioceptive and sensory input as a protective mechanism to restrain use of the threatened muscle or part. It may occur as the result of (1) altered sensory or proprioceptive input from any cause, e.g., altered dentition, dental treatment, local anesthesia, or unusual jaw position or movement; (2) volitional jaw movements that conflict with preexisting habit patterns or that arise from oral consciousness; (3) injury or threat of injury, strain, abusive use, or muscle fatigue; and (4) increased bruxism associated with emotional tension or illness.

Muscle splinting occurs insidiously but becomes symptomatic rapidly. Normally it is of short duration, lasting only a few days, and tends to disappear quickly when the etiologic factors resolve. Abusive use or injudicious therapy, however, may protract the splinting effect, which can terminate in myospasm. The clinical effects of muscle splinting are observed chiefly in the elevator muscles. On some occasions, the lateral pterygoid muscles may be involved, and myospasm can develop if such splinting is protracted.

SYMPTOMS.—The identifying characteristics by which masticatory muscle splinting can be recognized are:

1. History of recent prior altered sensory input, unusual jaw use, volitional chewing, minor strain, muscle fatigue, emotional crisis, illness, or dental treatment, especially if a local anesthetic has been used.

2. The pain is myogenous and of the muscle-splinting variety. It emanates from the splinted muscle and occurs especially when that muscle is contracted (chewing strokes with elevator muscles, opening against resistance with lateral pterygoid muscles). Muscle weakness may also be sensed.

3. No restriction of jaw movement is present except insofar as it is inhibited by the influence of pain or sensation of muscular weakness.

4. No interference during mandibular movement is evident.

5. No acute malocclusion is present.

6. No radiographic confirmation is available.

TABLE 8–3.—SYMPTOMS OF ACUTE MUSCLE DISORDERS

	MUSCLE SPLINTING	MASTICATORY PAIN-DYSFUNCTION SYNDROMES			MUSCLE INFLAMMATION
		SPASM OF ELEVATOR MUSCLE(S)	SPASM OF LATERAL PTERYGOID MUSCLE	SPASM OF ELEVATOR AND LATERAL PTERYGOID MUSCLES	
History	Prior altered sensory or proprioceptive input	Prior protracted muscle splinting, nonspastic myofascial pain syndrome, or other continuous deep pain input. Sustained high emotional stress, physical fatigue, or illness			Prior local muscle injury, infection, adjacent disease, or protracted MPD syndrome
Masticatory pain	Occurs with muscle contraction accompanied by muscle weakness	Occurs with opening and chewing. Not reduced by biting on a separator	Occurs with maximum intercuspation. Reduced by biting on a separator	Occurs with opening, chewing, and maximum intercuspation	Pain at rest and with all jaw use. Not reduced by biting on a separator
Restriction of movement	If any, due to inhibitory influence of pain and muscle weakness	Restricted opening due to spasm of elevator muscle or disc jamming	None	Restricted opening due to spasm of elevator muscle or disc jamming	Restricted opening due to swollen elevator muscle
Interference during movement	None	If any, due to increased interarticular pressure	If any, due to spastic lateral pterygoid muscle	If any, due to spastic elevator and lateral pterygoid muscles	None
Acute malocclusion	None	Minor malocclusion due to spastic elevator muscle	Gross malocclusion due to lateral pterygoid spasm	Gross malocclusion due to lateral pterygoid spasm	None
Radiographic confirmation	None	Positive for extracapsular restraint of condylar movement	Positive for gross malocclusion	Positive for extracapsular restraint of condylar movement and gross malocclusion	Positive for extracapsular restraint of condylar movement

Masticatory Muscle Spasm (MPD Syndrome)

Muscle spasm is regarded *clinically* as a CNS-induced involuntary tonic contraction of a muscle(s). It may occur as the result of several conditions, such as (1) protracted muscle splinting from any of the causes mentioned above, (2) preexisting nonspastic myofascial pain syndrome (involving that muscle) from any of the causes discussed in chapters 4 and 6, (3) myospasm activity secondarily induced as a central excitatory effect from deep-pain input elsewhere in the trigeminal area or secondary to deep facial, glossopharyngeal, or cervical pain syndromes, and (4) systemic illness, emotional tension, physical fatigue, or as an extrapyramidal effect of certain medications.

When myospastic activity develops a component of pain, it becomes an independent self-perpetuating cycling myospasm, no longer dependent on any cause. *As such it can cycle indefinitely.*

Cycling myospastic activity involving the masticatory musculature was described first in 1956 by Schwartz,[10] who used the term *temporomandibular joint pain-dysfunction syndrome* to designate the condition and distinguish it from structural joint disease. His work is recognized as a major breakthrough in our understanding of temporomandibular disorders. Since then, much research has been directed at muscle dysfunction, almost to the disregard of masticatory biomechanics. In more recent years, the myofascial pain-dysfunction syndrome (MPD syndrome) involving the masticatory musculature as reported by Laskin,[6] Greene,[4] and many other workers has tended to overshadow other temporomandibular disorders that plague humanity.

A simple cycling spasm of a masticatory muscle should present no problem, diagnostic or therapeutic. Unfortunately, spastic activity of elevator muscles increases the passive interarticular pressure, thus altering or interfering with normal biomechanics of the joint. As such, it predisposes to discal interference during mandibular movements. Also, spastic activity in the lateral pterygoid muscle induces acute malocclusion, thus initiating a chain of masticatory problems that involve the joint proper and the musculature. Spastic activity occurring simultaneously in elevator and lateral pterygoid muscles predisposes to disc-condyle complex dysfunction as well. Therefore, it is the *secondary effects* of what initially may be a simple muscle problem that complicate the biomechanical functioning of the masticatory apparatus and cause management problems. This is sufficient reason to manage acute myospasms of masticatory muscles with dispatch.

It should be understood that what initially may be nothing more than a simple muscle disorder may *activate* an otherwise dormant nonsymptomatic temporomandibular disorder and, therefore, become the dominant etiologic factor in a considerably more serious masticatory problem. To treat such conditions effectively, it is necessary to distinguish between muscle disorders and the more serious structural disorders of the joint proper.[1] The secondary effects of cycling muscle spasm activity may present the real challenge to the therapist. *Myospastic activity in masticatory muscles may cycle indefinitely, especially if subjected to continued painful use or to injudicious therapy.* Protracted or abused myospasm may develop into an inflammatory condition, myositis.

SYMPTOMS.—A myofascial pain-dysfunction syndrome usually is associated with a history of (1) protracted muscle splinting from any cause, (2) nonspastic myofascial pain syndrome involving a masticatory muscle, (3) some preexistent deep-pain input in the vast trigeminal area, or in the facial, glossopharyngeal, or cervical regions, (4) a period of high emotional stress, physical fatigue, or illness, or (5) medication with a tranquillizer such as phenothiazine.

Other identifying characteristics of masticatory myospasm disorders depend on which muscle(s) is involved and to what degree, as follows.

Spasm of Elevator Muscle(s).

1. The pain is myogenous and of the muscle-spasm variety. It emanates from the involved elevator muscle(s) when contracted (chewing) or stretched (opening). The chewing pain is not reduced by biting against a separator. (Note: If interarticular pressure increases sufficiently to induce some discal interference, associated intermittent disc-attachment arthralgic pain may be present also.)

2. Restriction of mandibular movement is extracapsular in type, thus causing restriction of opening only. Other movements may be inhibited by the influence of pain. (Note: If discal interference is sufficient to induce actual locking of the articular disc, intracapsular restriction of mandibular movement may occur also.)

3. No interference during mandibular movements occurs *unless* the spasm increases the passive interarticular pressure sufficiently to induce discal interference.

4. Acute malocclusion, if any, is minor and usually subjective.

5. Radiography may confirm extracapsular restriction of mandibular movement, with condylar movement in open position being definitely less than in lateral position.

Spasm of Lateral Pterygoid Muscle(s).

1. The pain is myogenous and emanates from the lateral pterygoid muscle when stretched (maximum intercuspation) or contracted (opening against resistance). The maximum-intercuspation pain is reduced by biting against a separator.

2. No restriction of mandibular movement is present.

3. Spastic muscle may impair disc-condyle complex functioning.

4. Acute malocclusion is observed as protrusion of the condyle (disocclusion of the ipsilateral posterior teeth and premature striking of the contralateral anterior teeth) due to the shortened muscle.

5. Radiography may confirm gross malocclusion, with the condyle in unclenched closed position being anterior to the clenched occluded position of the joint.

Spasm of Elevator and Lateral Pterygoid Muscles.

1. The pain is myogenous and emanates from both elevator and lateral pterygoid muscles when these are contracted or stretched (as on opening, chewing, or maximum intercuspation). The maximum-intercuspation pain may be reduced, but not eliminated, by biting against a separator. (Note: If much discal interference is present, some associated intermittent disc-attachment arthralgic pain may also be present.)

2. Restriction of mandibular movement is extracapsular, thus causing restriction of opening only. Other movements may be inhibited by the influence of pain. (Note: If discal interference is sufficient to induce locking of the articular disc, intracapsular restriction of mandibular movement may be present also.)

3. No interference during mandibular movement occurs unless the spasm increases the passive interarticular pressure sufficiently to cause discal interference.

4. Acute malocclusion is due to protrusion of the condyle (disocclusion of the ipsilateral posterior teeth and premature striking of the contralateral anterior teeth).

5. Radiography may confirm extracapsular restriction of mandibular movement, with condylar movement in open position being definitely less than in lateral position. Gross malocclusion may be observed, the condyle in unclenched closed position being anterior to the clenched occluded position of the joint.

Masticatory Muscle Inflammation (Myositis)

Inflammation of a masticatory muscle is regarded *clinically* as a localized reaction in the muscle in response to (1) local injury from such causes as unaccustomed or abusive use, strain, infection, and adjacent disease, (2) direct extension of inflammation from another inflammatory condition in a nearby structure, or (3) protracted or abused (injudiciously treated) myospastic activity from any of many possible causes.

SYMPTOMS.—The symptoms are those of an inflammatory condition and reflect the type, degree, and phase of inflammatory reaction present. The symptoms tend to follow an inflammatory curve in incidence, development, plateauing, and resolution. Generally, alteration in function outlasts pain as resolution takes place. Protracted myositis predisposes to muscular contracture of the myofibrotic kind. Clinically, myositis involves the elevator muscles chiefly. It tends to induce some associated secondary muscle splinting effects also.

The identifying characteristics of masticatory myositis are:

1. History of prior local injury, unaccustomed use, infection, adjacent disease, nearby inflammatory condition, or preexistent protracted myofascial pain-dysfunction syndrome.

2. The pain is myogenous and of the local muscle soreness variety. It emanates from the inflamed muscle and occurs when the muscle is at rest as well as with all masticatory use. The maximum-intercuspation pain is not reduced by biting against a separator. (Note: If secondary muscle splinting occurs, minor myogenous pain may be felt in other masticatory muscles with chewing efforts.)

3. Restriction of mandibular movement is extracapsular, thus restricting opening only. Other movements may be restrained by the inhibitory influence of pain.

4. No interference during mandibular movements is evident.

5. No acute malocclusion is present unless the lateral pterygoid muscle is involved.

6. Radiography confirms extracapsular restriction of mandibular movement, with condylar movement in the open position being definitely less than in the lateral position.

DISC-INTERFERENCE DISORDERS OF THE JOINT

Disorders due to interference with normal functioning of the articular disc occupy a position among temporomandibular complaints second only to the acute muscle disorders in incidence. In fact, if nonsymptomatic conditions of the masticatory apparatus are included, interference disorders of the joint no doubt rank first. This group includes particularly the noisy, clicking, popping joints, with or without a component of pain.

The term sometimes used to designate such complaints is "degenerative joint disease." It is satisfactory only if it is clearly understood that these conditions represent the noninflammatory phase of degenerative joint disease, not true inflammatory degenerative arthritis. In recent years such conditions have been referred to as internal derangements of the joint. They are morphofunctional disorders of the disc-condyle complex.

Disorders of this sort are grouped together because they have clinical features that are similar, and they appear to be related in that they frequently represent a progressive series of deleterious changes of the joint. Pain may or may not accompany the masticatory dysfunction symptoms that dominate the clinical symptom picture.

Extrinsic trauma may damage the joint proper. Violent injury, including fracture and fracture-dislocation, may result in structural disorders such as deformation, chronic mandibular hypomobility, or traumatic arthritis. Less severe trauma may cause capsulitis or retrodiscitis. Such sequelae to extrinsic trauma will be considered later. But, minor external trauma may initiate deleterious changes in the joint surfaces, e.g., a moderate blow to the mandible *when the teeth are separated* may damage the articular surface at some point along the articular eminence, thus causing the articulating parts to hang as they pass over the site of damage. Trauma sustained *when the teeth are occluded* may likewise damage the articular surface at the closed relationship of the joint, thus causing resistance to movement of the articular disc from the closed-joint position, especially after maximum intercuspation or following periods of inactivity. Damage may also be sustained by components of the disc-condyle complex—the collateral discal ligaments, the retrodiscal tissue, or the articular disc proper.

More frequently, the initiating factor that leads to interference disorders of the joint has to do with *microtraumas* sustained by the articulating parts of the joint as a result of structural or functional incompatibilities. Insidious damage may result from the habitual use of excessive biting force. It may relate to abusive habits, mannerisms, or use of the mouth and jaws for special purposes other than talking and mastication. But the most important parafunctional abuse no doubt relates to bruxism, both static and moving. In either case, the decisive factor that most significantly predisposes to deleterious change is occlusal disharmony—lack of functional compatibility between the muscle-induced, unclenched, closed-joint position and the clenched position of maximum intercuspation dictated solely by the inclined planes of occluded teeth. The primary activating factor that causes all such microtraumas to become potentially damaging to the joint is excessive passive interarticular pressure sustained by the joint, especially as it relates to increased emotional tension and bruxism. An important clinical feature common to interference disorders of the joint is intermittency.

The similarities by which interference disorders of the joint are grouped together are as follows:

1. Noninflammatory dysfunction symptoms dominate the complaints. These are interferences during movements expressed as sensations, noises, and alterations of movement. If any restriction of mandibular movement occurs, it is due to associated jamming of or blockage by the articular disc.

2. Pain, if any, relates to discal interference or jamming. It is disc-attachment arthralgia that results from strain or injury involving the collateral

ligaments as they offer resistance to the interference. Being intermittent, it does not tend to induce secondary central excitatory effects.

Chronic interference disorders of the joint do not induce muscle splinting or myospasm activity in the masticatory muscles. However, a recently instituted occlusal disharmony (e.g., from recent change in the dentition due to trauma, extraction of teeth, or dental treatment) or recent activation of a preexisting but nonsymptomatic interference disorder (as a result of abuse or excessive passive interarticular pressure, as from an emotional crisis or an episode of oral consciousness) may institute muscle splinting and, if protracted, develop into myospastic activity. When an acute muscle disorder initially complicates a disc-interference disorder, it is a good assumption that the interference disorder preexisted and was activated into a symptomatic complaint. If, however, the symptoms of interference follow in the wake of protracted myospasm, one may assume that deleterious change is taking place in the joint as a direct result of the myospastic activity. When acute muscle symptoms subsequently occur during a prolonged period of disc-interference symptoms, it may be assumed that the condition has progressed to the inflammatory stage, and that the muscle symptoms represent the effect of central hyperexcitability due to continuous deep-pain input.

Disc-interference disorders may become inflammatory. When this occurs, the condition should be reclassified as an *inflammatory disorder of the joint*. If arthralgic pain becomes constant, it may be identified as capsulitis, retrodiscitis, or inflammatory arthritis, depending on which structure is predominantly involved.

Interference disorders of the temporomandibular joint are classified according to how the symptoms of discal interference relate to the translatory cycle (see chap. 7). They are (1) Class I disorders, which occur before the cycle begins, (2) Class II disorders, which occur as the cycle begins or ends, (3) Class III disorders, which occur during the course of a normal cycle, (4) Class IV disorders, which occur when the cycle is extended beyond the normal anterior limits, and (5) spontaneous anterior dislocation, which occurs after termination of the translatory cycle anteriorly (Table 8–4).

Class I Interference

The symptoms of this class of interference occur in the closed position of the joint. They relate to maximum intercuspation of the teeth. The basic cause of this disorder is chronic occlusal disharmony of a kind and magnitude that displaces the disc-condyle complex from the unclenched closed position when the teeth are brought into maximum intercuspation. The condition that results depends on the degree, direction, duration, and fre-

TABLE 8–4.—SYMPTOMS OF DISC-INTERFERENCE DISORDERS OF THE JOINT

	CLASS I INTERFERENCE	CLASS II INTERFERENCE	CLASS III INTERFERENCE	CLASS IV INTERFERENCE	SPONTANEOUS ANTERIOR DISLOCATION
History	Persistent chronic occlusal disharmony	Persistent Class I interference Bruxism, habitual abusive use, or trauma	Increased interarticular pressure Persistent Class I or II interference Abusive use, trauma, or malocclusion	Habitually opening the mouth widely	Follows an excessively wide mouth opening
Masticatory pain	If any, at maximum intercuspation; reduced by biting on separator	If any, follows maximum intercuspation; reduced by preventing fully occluded joint position	If any, occurs with disc interference	If any, occurs with opening mouth widely	If any, occurs with forced reduction; may also have capsular or muscular pain
Restriction of movement	None	None	If any, due to jamming or dislocation of articular disc	None	Dislocated disc blocks closure of mouth
Interference during movement	Occurs with or immediately after maximum intercuspation Reduced by biting on separator	Follows maximum intercuspation or after protracted inactivity Reduced by preventing fully occluded joint position	Depends on cause: increased interarticular pressure; structural incompatibility; disrupted disc-condyle complex function	Occurs when mouth is opened widely	Arrested closure of mouth
Acute malocclusion	None	None	If any, due to fracture or dislocation of articular disc	None	Striking of posterior teeth with anterior open-bite
Radiographic confirmation	May be positive for gross malocclusion	May be positive for gross malocclusion	May be positive for change in width of disc space or subarticular bone	None	Positive for gross dislocation

quency of such abnormal movement. Any movement of the disc-condyle complex under frictional stress is potentially damaging to the articular surfaces and may provoke deleterious change in them.

If such disharmony has been created recently, as with changes in the dentition from trauma, extraction of posterior teeth, or dental treatment, an acute muscle disorder is more likely to result. Likewise, if a preexistent, dormant, nonsymptomatic, chronic occlusal disharmony is activated by bruxism due to an emotional crisis or by a period of oral consciousness, an acute muscle disorder may result. All such recently activated occlusal disharmony relates more closely to masticatory muscle spasm activity (MPD syndromes) than to the more subtle, less dramatic complaints that comprise disc-interference disorders.

SYMPTOMS.—The typical symptoms of Class I interference are a sensation of tightness or movement when the teeth are firmly clenched, frequently accompanied by momentary sharp pain, and then a discrete clicking sound just as the biting pressure is released. These symptoms can be prevented by biting ipsilaterally on a separator.

The identifying characteristics of Class I interference disorders are:

1. History of preexistent chronic occlusal disharmony.

2. Pain, if any, is disc-attachment arthralgia. It occurs intermittently as maximum intercuspation takes place and is reduced by biting against a separator.

3. No restricton of mandibular movement is observed.

4. Interference symptoms (abnormal sensation and noise) occur as the teeth are firmly clenched, or just as they are released. This is reduced by biting against a separator.

5. No *acute* malocclusion is present.

6. Radiographic confirmation of condylar displacement due to chronic occlusal disharmony is available if the displacement is gross enough and takes place in the sagittal plane. This is done by comparing the unclenched and clenched occluded positions of the joint (see Figs 7–8 and 7–9).

This type of discal interference predisposes to and may develop into a clinically identifiable Class II disc-interference disorder. Class I interference also predisposes to deleterious changes in the disc-condyle complex and as such may develop progressively into a Class III disc-interference disorder. Transitional phases between different classes of interference disorders may be difficult to define clinically. If such differentiation can be made, clinical management of the complaint is facilitated. It should be understood, however, that although etiologic factors responsible for Class I interference disorders may be reversible, the damage thus sustained by the joint structures may not be. *This is sufficient reason to understand and*

*identify disc-interference disorders at their earliest stage of development,
so that more recalcitrant conditions are avoided.*

Class II Interference

The symptoms of Class II disc-interference disorders occur immediately
following maximum intercuspation and as the translatory cycle begins.
Some interference may also be discerned when a power stroke ends in
maximum intercuspation. The noise initially emitted is usually a discrete
click and may be accompanied by momentary discomfort. A similar symptom may occur with the first movement following an extended period of
inactivity, especially if bruxism has taken place. The symptoms of this type
of interference can be prevented by inserting an occlusal stop between the
teeth to keep the disc-condyle complex from returning to its full, normal
closed-joint position.

Although Class II interference frequently develops from Class I interference as the result of chronic occlusal disharmony, it may stem from other
causes and present as a separate entity. Perhaps the most frequent cause
for this is trauma sustained when the teeth are occluded. Other factors may
be habitual use of excessive biting force and bruxism in the absence of
gross occlusal disharmony.

SYMPTOMS.—The identifying characteristics of Class II interference disorders of the joint are:

1. History of preexistent Class I interference disorder, prior trauma sustained when the teeth were occluded, bruxism, or habitual, excessively
hard biting and chewing.

2. Pain, if any, is disc-attachment arthralgia. It occurs intermittently in
association with the disc noise and can be prevented by inserting an occlusal stop between the teeth.

3. No restriction of mandibular movement is observed.

4. The interference occurs as a distinct click as the mouth is opened. It
follows maximum intercuspation or an extended period of inactivity. Firmly
clenching the teeth and then opening help to identify the typical symptoms. Separation of the teeth may reach 8 to 10 mm before the interference
occurs. Some modified interference may also be heard or sensed at the end
of the translatory cycle, *if a power stroke terminates in maximum intercuspation.* The symptoms can be prevented by inserting an occlusal stop between the teeth to keep the disc-condyle complex from returning to the
normal fully occluded position.

5. No *acute* malocclusion is present.

6. Radiographic confirmation may identify gross occlusal disharmony in

the sagittal plane. Destructive change sufficient to affect the subarticular bone sometimes may be evident radiographically.

Class II interference places considerable strain on the discal ligaments and, therefore, predisposes to Class III interference disorders as deterioration, elongation, or detachment of those ligaments takes place. The transitional phase may be difficult to identify when functional displacement of the disc occurs as the result of deterioration in the articular disc in conjunction with elongation of the discal ligaments.

Class III Interference

Symptoms of Class III disc-interference disorders occur during the course of normal translatory cycles— *after it begins, but not including strained movements or overextended opening.* Symptoms that occur as a result of forced, strained, or otherwise unnatural joint function are irrelevant to diagnosis.

Interference during translatory cycles may result from catching of the articular disc between the condyle and eminence. The result of such interference may be arrested movement. The inclination of the articular eminence should be considered, since the steeper the joint, the greater the likelihood of discal interference, and therefore the greater the importance of other factors that predispose to such interference.

Class III interference disorders occur for three basic reasons, namely, (1) excessive passive interarticular pressure, (2) lack of compatibility in the shape of the articulating surfaces, so that they hang as they glide over each other, and (3) some derangement or impairment of function involving the disc-condyle complex. Each of these will be considered etiologically and symptomatically.

EXCESSIVE PASSIVE INTERARTICULAR PRESSURE.—The passive interarticular pressure in the joint reflects muscle action. Minimal passive interarticular pressure is that exerted by muscle tonus as affected by negative gravity. Active interarticular pressure depends on the demands of function as affected by muscle contraction, resistance, torque, etc.

Passive interarticular pressure is increased by emotional tension and by spasm of elevator muscles. Excessive passive pressure is an activating factor in all other causes of discal interference, sometimes making symptomatic a condition that otherwise might remain quite dormant. Discal interference due to this cause may show variability and, sometimes, a pattern of recurrence that parallels the rise and fall of emotional tension.

STRUCTURAL INCOMPATIBILITY OF THE SLIDING SURFACES.—Structural incompatibility between the articulating surfaces (articular eminence and upper surface of the disc-condyle complex) sufficient to cause catching of the articular disc during translatory cycles may result from several causes. These include developmental anomalies, growth aberrations, trauma, remodeling, and change due to such things as abusive use, mannerisms, chronic occlusal disharmony, and unusual functional demands. Trauma to the mandible sustained when the teeth are separated is a frequent cause. Immobilization of the opposite joint for any reason causes movements that may induce destructive change within the joint. All such interference due to structural incompatibility relates intimately to the degree of passive interarticular pressure as well as to the speed and force of movement.

Interference due to this cause has a pattern of sameness and chronicity unless varying interarticular pressure gives it an episodic quality. Due to the sameness of behavior, interference of this type may be compensated for by deviation of the midline incisal path, considered to be an attempt on the part of muscles to find a way around the interference. When rapid movements are made, however, the initiating interference usually will become evident. Interference from structural incompatibility is less pronounced on the biting side during power strokes. This, together with deviation of the incisal path, is usually sufficient to identify it.

IMPAIRED DISC-CONDYLE COMPLEX FUNCTION.—The more recalcitrant and refractory Class III interferences occur as a result of functional impairment of the disc-condyle complex during otherwise normal translatory cycles and power strokes. Malfunctioning of the complex may be due to different structural abnormalities that result from chronic occlusal disharmony, trauma, or abusive use. These changes include (1) arrested hinge movement between the articular disc and mandibular condyle, (2) deterioration or fracture of the articular disc, (3) deterioration, elongation, or detachment of the discal ligaments, and (4) dysfunction of the superior retrodiscal lamina. Interference from such causes is usually progressive, thus predisposing to inflammatory degenerative arthritis. The particular structural problem represented by a given complaint may not be clearly discernible diagnostically because of transitional phases and the various possible combinations that can occur. It is important, however, that Class III interference from structural failure of disc-condyle complex functioning be identified, at least broadly, because such judgment is necessarily the basis for choosing a treatment modality for managing the complaint.

Adhesions Between the Articular Disc and Condyle.—Hemarthrosis induced by trauma may cause fibrous adhesions that unite the condylar articular facet with the lower surface of the articular disc. The elimination of hinge movement in the disc-condyle complex disrupts normal joint functioning during translatory movements. Smooth, silent, surface-to-surface gliding of the articular disc along the articular eminence is impossible, and such movement becomes a bodily skidding of the immobilized disc. The result is rough, irregular, noisy movement throughout all translatory cycles.

Damaged Articular Disc.—Roughening of the superior surface of the articular disc due to trauma or deleterious change provokes interference throughout the translatory cycle. This is manifested as a more or less continuous grating noise punctuated at points of greater resistance by discrete noise and sensations of catching. Such interference may increase during a power stroke, *if it is on the nonbiting side*. Thinning of the disc due to continuing destructive change may result in perforation. This may alter internal hydrodynamic action of the synovial fluid, about which little is presently known. Thinning also predisposes to disc fracture. Separated fragments of a fractured disc lead to acute malocclusion, sensed as overstressed posterior teeth during maximum intercuspation. Overriding fragments cause acute malocclusion, manifested as disocclusion of the posterior teeth. When the thinning occurs primarily in the normally thicker anterior or posterior portions of the articular disc, especially important disruption may occur in disc-condyle complex functioning. (Since such destructive change occurs in conjunction with deterioration and elongation of discal collateral ligaments, it will be considered in the following section.)

Dysfunctional Discal Ligaments.—The discal collateral ligaments that firmly attach the articular disc to the medial and lateral poles of the mandibular condyle are the essential structures that make the disc and condyle into a functioning hinge-joint unit—the disc-condyle complex. When the functional capability of these ligaments is compromised by deterioration, elongation, or detachment, normal hinge movement in the complex is lost, and sliding movement between the condyle and articular disc can take place. When the disc fails to follow the condyle closely, its essential function of maintaining sharp surface contact between the moving parts is impaired. It tends to catch and hang, thus causing irregular, rough, noisy movements. Discrete noises, catching sensations, and disc locking may take place. Noise and other symptoms of discal interference are likely to occur at the beginning of a power stroke when the superior lateral pterygoid muscle suddenly overcomes the posterior traction of the superior retrodiscal lamina. All such interference is particularly sensitive to other contributing factors, such as steepness of the articular eminence, excessive interarticular pressure, structural incompatibility, and speed and force of jaw movement.

Two kinds of Class III disorders that involve dysfunctional discal ligaments in conjunction with thinning of the anterior or posterior portions of the articular disc are functional displacements and functional dislocations of the articular disc.

Functional Displacement of the Disc.—The sequence of clicking, popping, or snapping noises emitted by the disc-condyle complex during opening and closing depends on the *location of destructive change* in the articular disc, the *extent of elongation* of discal ligaments, and the *kind of movements* made. Thinning of the posterior portion of the disc permits functional displacement in an anterior direction; thinning of the anterior portion permits displacement posteriorly. The extent of elongation of the discal ligaments determines the amount of displacement possible. The kind of mandibular movement as it relates to action of the superior lateral pterygoid muscle and the superior retrodiscal lamina determines the incidence of displacement.

1. *Posteriorly thinned articular disc.* In the occluded position, the articular disc is displaced anteriorly by action of the superior lateral pterygoid muscle. As the mouth is opened, the condyle moves forward over the displaced disc until it meets the thicker anterior portion, by which the disc is then moved forward also. Some minor disc noise may occur. The disc remains centered on the condyle until displaced anteriorly again by the superior lateral pterygoid muscle as the result of a power stroke, rapid closure, or return to the closed position, thus emitting discal noise.

2. *Anteriorly thinned articular disc.* After maximum intercuspation, the disc may remain against the articular fossa as the condyle begins to move forward. When the limit of the elongated discal ligaments is reached, the disc is dislodged and brought back to its condylar position by the extended (not contracted) superior lateral pterygoid muscle, thus emitting discal noise. As translatory movement continues, the disc is again displaced posteriorly by the extended superior retrodiscal lamina. Then, contraction of the superior lateral pterygoid muscle replaces the disc to its condylar position as the result of a power stroke, rapid closure, or return to the closed position, thus emitting discal noise.

During functional displacements of the articular disc, *momentary or protracted disc jamming* may take place. Although displacement from its normal position occurs, the disc is not dislocated from the condyle. It still remains in firm contact between the condyle and articular eminence.

Functional Dislocation of the Disc.—If elongation, deterioration, or detachment of the discal collateral ligaments progresses until still greater displacement is permitted, and if deterioration of the articular disc is such as to permit it to be pulled through the articular disc space, functional dislocation of the disc can take place. There are different kinds of dislocation of the disc, namely, (1) spontaneous dislocation, which occurs with overextended opening and takes place in an anterior direction only, (2) traumatic dislocation, which results from direct external force (violence), and (3) functional dislocation, which occurs during the *normal* functioning of the joint and within the normal range of movement. Functional dislocation occurs as the result of structural abnormality in the disc-condyle complex. When this happens, contact between condyle, disc, and articular eminence is lost, the articular disc space collapses, and the disc becomes trapped (in front of or behind the condyle, as the case may be).

1. *Anterior functional dislocation of the disc* can occur when there is sufficient deterioration of the posterior portion of the articular disc to permit it to be pulled through the articular disc space anteriorly. The force that causes dislocation is contraction of the superior lateral pterygoid muscle during a power stroke, rapid closure, or maximum intercuspation. *It is more likely to occur on the biting side due to widening of the articular disc space.* The dislocation is manifested by discrete discal noise. When the articular disc space collapses, the disc is trapped anterior to the condyle, where it remains until automatically reduced by posterior traction of the superior retrodiscal lamina as a full forward translatory movement is executed. At that time, discal noise is again emitted as reduction of the dislocation takes place. It should be noted, however, that if the dislocated disc should block normal anterior movement of the condyle, then functional reduction is impossible, and the dislocated condition of the articular disc becomes protracted.

2. *Posterior functional dislocation of the disc* can occur when there is sufficient deterioration of the anterior portion of the articular disc to permit it to be pulled through the articular disc space posteriorly. The force that causes such dislocation is the posterior traction of the extended superior retrodiscal lamina during a full forward translatory cycle. The dislocation is manifested by discrete discal noise. When the articular disc space collapses, the disc is trapped posterior to the condyle until automatically reduced by the next closing effort, the reduction being accomplished by contraction of the superior lateral pterygoid muscle as the result of a power stroke, rapid closure, or intercuspation. Discal noise is again heard as reduction takes place. Protracted posterior functional dislocation does not occur.

The timing of the discal interference characteristic of functional dislocations depends on the actual mandibular movements made, as they relate to action of the superior lateral pterygoid muscle and the superior retrodiscal lamina, *for these are the forces that cause the dislocations and effect reduction as well.* Between dislocation and reduction, movements are rough and noisy in the absence of a functioning disc.

Dysfunctional Superior Retrodiscal Lamina.—Although the width of the articular disc space as determined by interarticular pressure is the final determinant of the exact rotatory position of the articular disc on the mandibular condyle (see chap. 3), other influencing factors are essential to ensure proper joint stability. The collateral ligaments keep the parts of the disc-condyle complex in a close hinge-joint relationship. The superior lateral pterygoid muscle passively maintains an anterior rotatory position of the disc when the joint is at rest and actively rotates the disc forward during power strokes and maximum intercuspation. The superior retrodiscal lamina rotates the articular disc posteriorly during the forward phase of the translatory cycle, thus supplying the joint with stability during the critical turn-around maneuver as the return phase of the translatory cycle begins. During empty-mouth cycles, there is a shift from anterior to posterior rotatory influence on the disc during the forward movement and a similar shift from posterior to anterior rotatory influence during the return phase. This is accomplished by the gradually increasing posterior traction created by the stretching elastic superior retrodiscal lamina during the forward phase, and a decreasing effect as it relaxes during the return phase. Normal functioning of this elastic retrodiscal structure is essential to smooth, silent functioning of the disc-condyle complex.

If the superior retrodiscal lamina is severed from the articular disc as a result of trauma, there is anterior prolapse of the disc to the extent permitted by the width of the articular disc space. This is manifested by discal interference consisting of rough, irregular, noisy movements, especially during the forward turn-around phase of translatory cycles. The danger of spontaneous anterior dislocation is greatly increased, and if it should occur, it is permanent because no other joint structure can be manipulated to exert posterior traction on the articular disc and thus bring about reduction.

Likewise, if conditions are such as to permit functional dislocation of the articular disc, as discussed above, and if such dislocation should occur in an anterior direction, it is irreversible except by surgical intervention.

SYMPTOMS.—The clinical manifestations of Class III interference are varied and numerous. In general, the identifying characteristics include:

1. History of cause for increased interarticular pressure; preexistent Class I or II interference disorders; or alterations in the disc-condyle complex functioning due to trauma, abusive use, or chronic occlusal disharmony.

2. Masticatory pain, *if any,* is arthralgic disc-attachment pain that occurs in conjunction with the symptoms of interference.

3. Restriction of mandibular movement, if any, is intracapsular and due to disc jamming or blockage of condylar movement by an anteriorly dislocated articular disc.

4. Interference during mandibular movement depends on increased passive interarticular pressure, structural incompatibility of the sliding surfaces, deterioration or fracture of the articular disc, arrested movement between the disc and condyle, dysfunctional discal ligaments, or a dysfunctional superior retrodiscal lamina. Interference includes rough, irregular, noisy movements punctuated by discrete noises and interference with movement, deviations of the midline incisal path, disc locking, and blocked movement.

5. Acute malocclusion consists of a sensation of overstressed posterior teeth in maximum intercuspation when fragments of a fractured articular disc are separated or when the disc is dislocated from the condyle. If fragments of a fractured disc override, disocclusion of the posterior teeth is sensed.

6. Radiographic confirmation may indicate gross occlusal disharmony (if it occurs in the sagittal plane), gross osseous changes in the subarticular bone, and arrested condylar movement.

Note should be taken of the diagnostic and therapeutic importance of properly identifying the different kinds of intracapsular restriction of mandibular movement due to jamming or dislocation of the articular disc. This can be done by observing the following clinical criteria:

Acute disc jamming (functional discal ligaments)
> Momentary: Disc-attachment pain if forced
>> Disc noise is emitted when jamming is relieved by manipulation
> Protracted: Increasing pain (acute discitis and eventually capsulitis)
>> Discal noise and pain when jamming is relieved
>> Restriction of protrusive and lateral movements also

Disc jamming due to dysfunctional discal ligaments (functional displacement)
> Momentary: Little or no pain sensed when forced
>> Minimal discal noise emitted when jamming is relieved by manipulation
> Protracted: Remains relatively painless
>> Movements within the range permitted are silent
>> No associated sensation of acute malocclusion during maximum intercuspation
>> Considerable protrusive or lateral movement permitted
>> Little or no noise or pain elicited when jamming is relieved by manipulation

Movement blocked by anteriorly dislocated disc (functional dislocatio)
> Momentary: Little or no pain sensed when forced

Released by manipulation, followed by opening the
mouth widely

Protracted: Becomes painful with symptoms of acute retrodiscitis

Movements within the range permitted are noisy and
grating

Acute malocclusion is sensed during maximum intercuspation (ipsilateral overstressed posterior teeth)

Restriction of protrusive and lateral movements also

Manipulation may or may not relieve the blockage

The following are clinical indications suggestive of Class III interference
disorders from different causes:

Due to excessive passive interarticular pressure:
Variability
Sudden onset and change
Recurrence and/or periodicity of symptoms

Due to structural incompatibility between the sliding surfaces:
Patterns of sameness and chronicity, unless varying passive interarticular pressure (due to rhythmic fluctuation of emotional tension)
gives it an episodic time frame

The presence of well developed deviations of the incisal path during
routine opening-closing movements

Evidence that symptoms are decreased by chewing on the symptomatic side

Due to impaired disc-condyle complex functioning:
Recalcitrant, progressive, and continuous symptoms, punctuated by
disc locking

Reciprocal functional displacements of the articular disc

Reciprocal functional dislocations of the articular disc

Sensation of acute malocclusion consisting of overstressed or disoccluded ipsilateral posterior teeth during maximum intercuspation

Evidence of protracted anterior dislocation of the articular disc

Evidence that symptoms are accentuated by chewing on the symptomatic side

Note should be taken of the therapeutic importance of precisely identifying functional dislocations of the articular disc. This is because surgical
intervention may be the treatment of choice in some cases, but not in
others. *It is important to be able to identify clinically which cases may
require a surgical approach.*

1. First, it is important to distinguish between anterior and posterior
functional dislocations of the articular disc. Anterior dislocations may re-

quire surgery; posterior dislocations usually do not.

Anterior dislocation occurs during a power stroke and is normally reduced during a full forward translatory movement. Thus, the symptoms of noise and interference occur first during a power stroke (usually on the biting side) and second during a full forward translatory cycle (opening widely). During the interval between symptoms, movement is rough and noisy, and acute malocclusion (overstressed ipsilateral posterior teeth) may be sensed during maximum intercuspation.

Posterior dislocation, in contrast, occurs during a full forward translatory cycle and normally is reduced during the closing movement. This occurs as a single opening-biting movement. Thus, the symptoms of noise and interference occur first with opening widely and second during the closing stroke.

The identifying difference, therefore, between anterior and posterior functional dislocation is the timing of the symptoms. Seldom is surgical intervention justified for complaints of this kind. Other means of management, the effectiveness of which depends largely on proper identification of the type of dislocation, are available.

2. Protracted functional dislocation of the articular disc is a different matter. It should be understood that *protracted posterior dislocation does not occur,* because nothing interferes with automatic functional reduction. Two conditions, however, may prevent automatic functional reduction of *anterior* dislocation, namely, (1) blockage of forward translatory movement by the dislocated and distorted disc, and (2) a nonfunctional superior retrodiscal lamina. It is important to distinguish between these two conditions. A blocked, dislocated disc may sometimes be manipulated without surgically opening the joint; the nonfunctional lamina will cause the disc to remain permanently dislocated without surgical intervention.

In both cases, all movements are rough and noisy, and acute malocclusion (overstressed ipsilateral posterior teeth) may be sensed during maximum intercuspation. Symptoms of retrodiscitis become evident. The identifying difference between the two conditions is the *extent of translatory movement.* When protracted anterior dislocation is due to a dislocated articular disc that blocks condylar movement, clinical and radiographic evidence of intracapsular restriction of mandibular movement is present. When the protracted dislocation is due to a nonfunctional superior retrodiscal lamina (usually the result of external trauma), the gross mandibular movements remain clinically and radiographically within the limits of normal.

Class IV Interference

Subluxation refers to partial or incomplete dislocation of the articulating surfaces of a joint. In the temporomandibular joint, this can occur when translatory movement takes place without benefit of rotatory movement between the condyle and articular disc. Such arrested hinge movement can occur if forward movement of the condyle exceeds that of the normal translatory cycle.

The forward limit of normal translatory movement is reached when the disc can no longer rotate posteriorly on the condyle, as determined by the condylar articular facet. As mouth opening takes place, the condyle rotates in the disc to separate the jaws and the disc rotates on the condyle to maintain surface contact with the articular eminence. When these combined movements bring the posterior edge of the articular disc to the posterior margin of the condylar articular facet, hinge movement is arrested. Further opening effort causes partial dislocation between the disc and articular eminence (see Fig 3–7). Such continued forward movement consists of a rough, jumping skid instead of smooth, silent, gliding, surface-to-surface movement of the disc-condyle complex along the temporal articular facet.

Class IV interference disorders occur *anterior to normal translation* due to excessive opening of the mouth, usually on a habitual level. Just prior to the typical jumping movement, a momentary pause usually is sensed. Then the condyle suddenly leaps forward to its full extent. The rough irregular movement is accompanied by noise and sometimes discomfort as well. Such interference does not take place in protrusive or lateral excursive movement because, without appreciable separation of the jaws, the limit of possible posterior rotation of the disc is not reached. This kind of disorder is usually referred to clinically as subluxation or joint hypermobility.

No doubt the development of muscular habit patterns that execute the subluxation movement is important in this complaint. Occasionally, oral conditions impose the need for excessive movement in the joints to open the mouth adequately. For example, overeruption and overlapping of the incisors may be so great as to require considerable separation of the jaws just to separate the teeth. Sufficient opening to accommodate the introduction of food into the mouth may entail excessive translatory movement in the joints. It should be noted that subluxation is more likely to occur with steeply inclined articular eminences. Subluxation predisposes to spontaneous anterior dislocation of the joint.

SYMPTOMS.—The identifying characteristics of Class IV interference disorders of the joint are:

1. History of excessive opening of the mouth, usually habitual.

2. Pain, if any, is disc-attachment arthralgia. It occurs intermittently with the dysfunction symptoms.

3. No restriction of mandibular movement is observed.

4. The interference occurs when the mouth is opened excessively. It

consists of a momentary pause, followed by a sudden irregular jumping forward of the condyle, accompanied by discal noise.

5. No acute malocclusion is present.

6. Radiographic confirmation is not available.

Spontaneous Anterior Dislocation

Normally, at the critical forward phase of the translatory cycle, sharp contact of the articulating parts is maintained by two conditions: (1) strong posteriorly directed rotatory traction on the articular disc exerted by the fully stretched superior retrodiscal lamina, and (2) relaxation of the superior lateral pterygoid muscle, so that no significant anteriorly directed counterforce is brought to bear on the disc. These conditions maintain a positive influence on the articular disc and, thus, preclude spontaneous dislocation. They keep it rotated as far posteriorly as the prevailing width of the articular disc space permits, thereby supplying continuing firm surface contact between the articulating parts.

Momentary muscular incoordination, however, can alter this protective relationship and induce dislocation. Normally, the superior lateral pterygoid muscle remains inactive throughout the translatory cycle, unless a power stroke ensues. Such strokes do not normally begin until after the forward turn-around phase of the cycle is completed and the return phase is well under way. Extremely precise timing of muscle action is required to accomplish this maneuver, especially when movements are rapid and when habitual subluxation presents an added hazard. If premature contraction of the superior lateral pterygoid muscle takes place at the full forward (or overextended) position of the disc-condyle complex, such muscle action immediately overcomes the posterior traction force of the stretched superior retrodiscal lamina; the articular disc is rotated anteriorly on the condyle; and spontaneous dislocation occurs (Figs 8–1 and 8–2). No doubt, this mechanism accounts for the occasional acute spontaneous anterior dislocation of the temporomandibular joints that occurs with yawning or when the muscles are fatigued by keeping the mouth open too long.

Another condition, however, is a frequent cause of spontaneous dislocation. This has to do with the biomechanics of the posterior capsular ligament. As the condyle moves forward, the loose accordion-like folds of the posterior portion of the capsular ligament open up and the capsule straightens out. At full forward position, the posterior capsular ligament may become taut (see Fig 3–7). When this occurs, further forward movement of the condyle cannot take place. Instead, it simply rotates on itself. If the articular disc is already rotated posteriorly to its full limit as determined by the condylar articular facet (see Fig 8–1), further rotatory movement of the

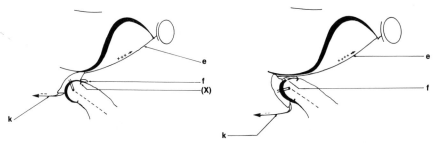

Fig 8–1.—Spontaneous anterior dislocation of disc-condyle complex: *e,* superior retrodiscal lamina; *f,* inferior retrodiscal lamina; *k,* superior lateral pterygoid muscle; *x,* posterior margin of condylar articular facet. *Left,* subluxated disc-condyle complex prior to dislocation. Articular disc is fully rotated posteriorly. Dominant traction force on disc is that of the stretched superior retrodiscal lamina. Disc-condyle complex rotates bodily upon itself. Superior lateral pterygoid muscle is inactive. *Right,* dislocated disc-condyle complex. When articular disc loses contact with the articular eminence, the disc space collapses, the condyle moves superiorly against the articular eminence, and the disc is trapped in front. During dislocation, the posterior traction force of the superior retrodiscal lamina continues to act on the articular disc at all times except when the superior lateral pterygoid muscle contracts in conjunction with elevator muscles in attempts to close the mouth. Note that the extent of forward rotatory prolapse of the articular disc during dislocation is limited by the inferior retrodiscal lamina. An attempt to force closure against the trapped disc may cause strain on this ligament.

condyle takes the disc with it and, thus, may push it through the articular disc space. When this happens, spontaneous anterior dislocation takes place. This mechanism very likely accounts for many such dislocations, especially those that recur frequently and can be executed almost at will.

In spontaneous anterior dislocation, the articular disc prolapses on the condyle (see Fig 8–2). Contact between condyle, disc, and eminence is lost. The articular disc space collapses and the condyle moves up against the eminence, thus trapping the disc anterior to the condyle. The amount of prolapse of the disc is limited by the inferior retrodiscal lamina, and attempts to close may stretch and cause undue strain on this ligamentous structure. Thus, forcing closure of the mouth without first reducing the dislocation may cause pain that emanates from the inferior retrodiscal lamina as well as the collateral discal ligaments.

It should be noted that the stretched superior retrodiscal lamina all the while is exerting positive posterior traction on the dislocated articular disc. This offers a ready means of spontaneous reduction, if only a sufficient width of articular disc space is provided to permit its return back to position on the condyle. This should be remembered as the key factor in planning treatment for this condition. Many patients who dislocate frequently

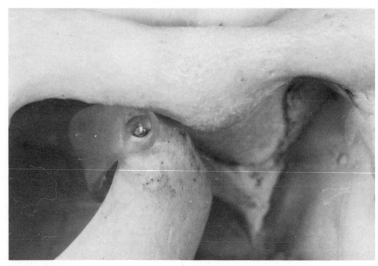

Fig 8–2.—Photograph of dry skull with simulated articular disc hinged on condyle to illustrate the disc-condyle relationship that prevails during spontaneous anterior dislocation. Note that articular disc is prolapsed anteriorly, articular disc space is collapsed, condyle is in contact with the articular eminence, and the prolapsed disc is trapped in front of the condyle.

learn to effect reduction of the disc automatically and can do so at will.

Spontaneous anterior dislocation is characterized by sudden inability to close the mouth following a wide opening effort. Only the most posteriorly located teeth come into contact while the anteriors stand widely apart. No pain is induced unless force is used to reduce the dislocation. Force may strain the inferior retrodiscal lamina, thus inducing arthralgic pain. Forced efforts to close the mouth also may injure the discal ligaments, thus causing symptoms of capsulitis. Myospastic activity in the musculature may add to the discomfort and the problem of reduction. Myospasm of the superior lateral pterygoid muscle prevents reduction entirely because it supercedes the ability of the superior retrodiscal lamina to reposition the disc, even if adequate disc space is provided. Contracture of this muscle causes chronic anterior dislocation. A nonfunctional superior retrodiscal lamina renders the dislocation permanent.

SYMPTOMS.—The identifying characteristics of spontaneous anterior dislocation are:

1. History of excessive opening of the mouth.
2. Masticatory pain, if any, is arthralgic and occurs as a result of forceful

reduction efforts. Traumatic reduction may cause capsulitis symptoms due to inflammation of the discal ligaments. Secondary myospasm pain may complicate the symptom picture.

3. Restriction of mandibular movement consists of inability to close the mouth properly from the wide-open position.

4. Interference during mandibular movement consists of arrested return phase of the translatory cycle due to blockage by the prolapsed articular disc.

5. Gross acute malocclusion consists of striking of the posterior teeth (or edentulous ridges) only, with the anteriors remaining widely apart.

6. Radiographic confirmation is available but unnecessary.

INFLAMMATORY DISORDERS OF THE JOINT

Inflammatory disorders of the joint have pain as their chief symptom— more or less continuous inflammatory arthralgic pain.[2] It tends to parallel the clinical course of the inflammatory process from which it emanates. Usually it is aggravated by the demands of function. Since it is usually continuous, secondary central excitatory effects are to be expected as part of the symptom complex.

The chief clinical features that cause these conditions to be grouped together for classification are:

1. History of trauma, infection, polyarthralgia, or noninflammatory degenerative condition of the joint.

2. More or less continuous arthralgia related to the demands of function, manual palpation of the joint proper, and functional manipulation.

3. Frequently complicated by referred pains, secondary hyperalgesia, and muscle-spasm activity in the masticatory muscles.

Inflammatory disorders of the temporomandibular joint may be classified as (1) synovitis and capsulitis, (2) retrodiscitis, and (3) inflammatory arthritis (Table 8–5).

Synovitis and Capsulitis

Inflammation of the synovial membrane and capsular ligament causes swelling and palpable tenderness over the involved joint. Synovitis proper characteristically causes fluctuating swelling due to effusion within the joint cavity, discomfort with joint movements, and alteration of the joint fluid. It may result from localized trauma, abusive use, and specific infection. Inflammation of the capsular ligament may result from several causes, namely, (1) strain or injury due to forced excessive condylar movement, (2) inflammatory condition of the discal collateral ligaments or the tempor-

TABLE 8–5.—SYMPTOMS OF INFLAMMATORY DISORDERS OF THE JOINT

	SYNOVITIS AND CAPSULITIS	RETRODISCITIS	INFLAMMATORY ARTHRITIS
History	Prior trauma Inflammation of discal ligaments or temporomandibular ligament Prior capsular fibrosis Periarticular inflammation	Prior recent trauma Activated preexistent nonanchored posterior overclosure	Prior trauma, infection, illness, progressive degenerative disorder, involvement of other joints, or arthropathy
Masticatory pain	Capsular type arthralgia Continuous but variable, increases with stretching of capsule Palpable tenderness over joint proper Secondary pains may occur	Retrodiscal type arthralgia Intermittent Occurs with maximum intercuspation Reduced by biting against a separator	Arthropathy type arthralgia Continuous but variable Relates to functional demands Usually accompanied by capsulitis Secondary pains may occur
Restriction of movement	Capsular type restrained joint movement Variable in degree, up to complete immobilization Extracapsular restraint due to secondary spasm	None	If any, due to capsulitis, preexistent disorder or arthropathy, or secondary myospasm activity
Interference during movement	If any, due to preexistent disorder	If any, due to preexistent disorder	If any, due to preexistent disorder
Acute malocclusion	If any, due to accumulation of intracapsular fluid	Posterior disocclusion with premature contact of contralateral anteriors	If any, due to intracapsular fluid, preexistent disorder or arthropathy, or secondary lateral pterygoid spasm
Radiographic confirmation	Positive for location of restricted movement and gross malocclusion	Positive for gross malocclusion	Positive for location of restricted movement, gross malocclusion, change in subarticular bone, or preexistent disorder or arthropathy

omandibular ligament, (3) inflammatory arthritis, (4) excessive condylar movement in the presence of preexisting capsular fibrosis, and (5) direct extension from a periarticular inflammatory process.

It is difficult, and indeed clinically impractical, to distinguish between synovitis and capsulitis. The identifying characteristics of synovitis and capsulitis are:

1. History of prior trauma or some preexisting condition that could secondarily involve the capsule in an inflammatory process.

2. Pain is more or less continuous and of the capsular arthralgic type. There is palpable tenderness over the joint proper, and the discomfort is increased by condylar movements that tend to stretch the capsule. (Note: If capsular pain increases in maximum intercuspation and is somewhat reduced by biting against a separator, the collateral ligaments and/or temporomandibular ligament should be suspected as the primary source of the inflammation.) Central excitatory effects may be seen also.

3. Restriction of mandibular movement, if any, is of capsular type. It may range from minor restriction of movement in the outer limits only to immobilization of the joint.

4. Usually, no interference during mandibular movement is present other than from a preexisting or coexisting condition. Sometimes gelation of the synovial fluid causes stiffness of the joint, especially after a period of inactivity. This may be accompanied by peculiar joint sounds. Such symptoms usually disappear rapidly as normal activity of the joint is reestablished.

5. Acute malocclusion, if any, is due to inflammatory effusion within the joint cavity, causing a sensation of disocclusion of the ipsilateral posterior teeth.

6. Radiography may confirm capsular restriction of mandibular movement (see Fig 7–6). Acute malocclusion, if any, may also be confirmed by comparing the width of the articular disc space in the unclenched and clenched occluded positions.

Retrodiscitis

Injury sustained by the retrodiscal tissues, either as a result of direct external trauma or due to condylar encroachment from any cause, may induce inflammation of the retrodiscal tissues, attended by intracapsular pain and swelling. Swelling of the tissue and effusion of inflammatory exudate in the joint cavity may displace the condyle anteriorly, thus causing acute malocclusion. This is sensed as disocclusion of the ipsilateral posterior teeth and premature striking of the contralateral anterior teeth. Pain occurs especially when maximum intercuspation forces the condyle back against the inflamed retrodiscal tissue. This pain can be reduced by biting against a separator to prevent intercuspation. Intermittency of the pain reduces the incidence of excitatory effects. Since the clinical symptoms of retrodiscitis in some ways simulate those of Class I interference, as well as spastic activity involving the lateral pterygoid muscle, careful differentiation is needed. If hemarthrosis takes place, ankylosis may result.

The identifying characteristics of retrodiscitis are:

1. History of extrinsic trauma, especially of the type that might have caused a mandibular fracture, if the condition is acute. Chronic retrodiscitis may relate to preexisting chronic occlusal or skeletal disharmonies or to protracted functional anterior dislocation.

2. Pain is arthralgic and of the retrodiscal variety. It is initiated or aggravated by maximum intercuspation of the teeth and reduced by a separator that prevents such intercuspation. Pain may be intermittent.

3. No restriction of mandibular movement is observed other than the inhibitory influence of pain.

4. No interference during mandibular movements is present other than preexisting symptoms.

5. Acute malocclusion is due to displacement of the condyle anteriorly as a result of swelling of the retrodiscal tissue or inflammatory effusion within the joint cavity. This is sensed as disocclusion of the ipsilateral posterior teeth and premature striking of the contralateral anteriors.

6. Acute malocclusion may be confirmed radiographically by comparing the unclenched and clenched occluded positions of the joint. The unclenched position shows the condyle to be anteriorly displaced.

Inflammatory Arthritis

Ordinarily, the clinical identification of intracapsular inflammation is sufficient to make a diagnosis of inflammatory arthritis. The complex structure and functional intricacies of the temporomandibular joints offer exceptions to this rule, as indicated by inflammatory conditions of the collateral ligaments, the temporomandibular ligaments, and the retrodiscal tissue. It is important therapeutically that clinical differentiation be made. It should be noted that capsulitis is frequently a feature of inflammatory arthritis.

The different types of inflammatory arthritis may be indistinguishable on the basis of clinical symptoms. The initial step is to establish with certainty that such a condition is present. The particular type can later be determined on the basis of etiology, clinical response to therapy, and laboratory studies.

The identifying characteristics of inflammatory arthritis are:

1. History of trauma, infection, systemic illness, involvement of other

joints, prior noninflammatory disc-interference disorder, ankylosis, or structural aberration.

2. Pain is arthralgic. Frequently, enough capsulitis is present to render the joint tender to manual palpation over the joint proper. Pain is more or less continuous but increases with functional demands. The symptom picture may be complicated by central excitatory effects. The speed and force of masticatory movements influence the discomfort.

3. Restriction of mandibular movement may be negligible. At other times, capsulitis and secondary muscle effects may immobilize the joint.

4. Interference during mandibular movement is consistent with preexisting etiologic conditions, such as a disc-interference disorder or trauma.

5. Acute malocclusion (other than that related to a preexisting condition) results from inflammatory effusion within the joint cavity. Some acute malocclusion may also be caused by lateral pterygoid muscle spasm as a secondary central excitatory effect.

6. Radiographic studies may be decisive, especially if the subarticular osseous structures are grossly involved. They may also confirm gross malocclusion and the location of restriction of mandibular movement, if such symptoms are clinically evident.

The pain level with different kinds of inflammatory arthritis is extremely variable. The same is true of functional interference. It may be surprising to see minimal pain and dysfunction when joint changes are great (e.g., some cases of degenerative arthritis). At other times, the discomfort may be wholly disproportionate to the structural change (e.g., hyperuricemia).

Different kinds of inflammatory arthritis afflict the temporomandibular joints, namely, traumatic arthritis, degenerative arthritis, infectious or septic arthritis, rheumatoid arthritis, and hyperuricemia.

TRAUMATIC ARTHRITIS.—Inflammatory arthritis that results from extrinsic trauma usually is expressed initially as a synovitis, with or without hemarthrosis. Other structures of the joint may suffer injury, e.g., the articular disc, collateral ligaments, retrodiscal tissue, and the osseous supported articular surfaces of the joint. Localized pain and swelling over the joint proper, discomfort with and restriction of joint function, and interference during joint movements may occur, depending on the location and extent of injury. Usually, single joints are involved. An important diagnostic clue is a history of continuity of symptoms from the time of trauma to the joint. Coexisting muscle effects should be recognized, such as splinting, spasm, or inflammation. Secondary central excitatory effects may also develop if the acute symptoms persist.

Radiographic studies may give evidence of traumatized osseous structures. Chronic forms of traumatic arthritis may show radiographic evidence of previous injury to the articular surfaces that cause interference with normal functioning of the joint (Fig 8–3).

DEGENERATIVE ARTHRITIS.—Degenerative arthritis is the advanced inflammatory phase of disc-interference disorders, as previously described. The history, therefore, is that of preexisting interference during mandibular movement. Although the examiner may not be able to discern the particular type of interference disorder represented, he may be able to identify etiologic factors that should be taken into consideration therapeutically. Chronic occlusal disharmony, especially aggravated by bruxism and activated by a high level of emotional tension, deserves careful consideration in all such conditions. The Class III disorders, especially those due to impaired disc-condyle complex function, predispose to inflammatory degenerative arthritis.

Although all sorts of functional abuse, including habitual excessive use of biting force, traumatic mannerisms and habits, nonphysiologic use of the mouth and jaws, bruxism, and occlusal interference of different kinds, are important etiologically in degenerative arthritis, one type of abusive force warrants special attention. That has to do with traumatic loading of the joint. Normally, joints are able to cope with considerable abuse and generally undergo various degrees and kinds of structural remodeling to compensate for conditions imposed on them. Overloading, however, tends to

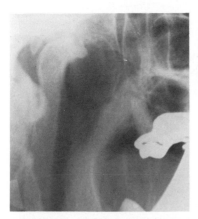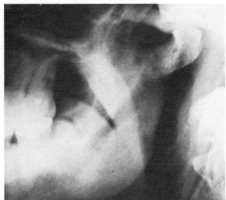

Fig 8–3.—Radiographic confirmation of traumatic arthritis. *Left,* transfacial projection of left mandibular condyle deformed as result of former injury. *Right,* transfacial projection of a fractured mandibular condyloid process that has healed in malposition. (Reproduced with permission from Bell W.E.: *Orofacial Pains: Differential Diagnosis,* ed. 2. Copyright © 1979 by Year Book Medical Publishers, Inc., Chicago.)

induce degenerative change in articular surfaces rather than physiologic remodeling.

When occlusal support in the posterior region of the mouth is insufficient, maximum intercuspation (clenching) causes the mandible to overclose in the posterior area—so-called posterior overclosure. If the remaining occluding teeth do not offer occlusal anchorage, the condyle slips posteriorly. But, if the remaining teeth do firmly hold the mandible and thus prevent posterior displacement, a fulcrum is formed at the location of the most posteriorly situated anchoring contact. Then, as the teeth are fully occluded, the condyle rotates around this fulcrum, and the excessive force generated by the overclosure is directed upward and forward into the articular eminence surface. Degenerative change is likely to take place in the impacted area as overloading occurs each time the teeth are brought into maximum intercuspation. Bruxism under these circumstances is especially abusive.

Radiographic confirmation of degenerative arthritis may include evidence of structural change in the subarticular bone (Fig 8–4). Evidence of occlusal disharmony also may be obtained if the disharmony is gross enough and takes place in the sagittal plane (see Figs 7–8 and 7–9).

INFECTIOUS ARTHRITIS.—Although synovitis may occur in conjunction with systemic infection as a nonspecific or immunologic response, actual purulent bacterial invasion of the joint may take place also. This may be due to penetrating wounds, trauma, or the spreading of infection from adjacent structures (e.g., otitis media). Occasionally, infectious arthritis may be the result of bacteremia from systemic infection (e.g., gonorrheal arthritis). The diagnosis is made from the history, clinical symptoms, examination of fluid aspirated from the joint cavity, and blood studies.[5]

RHEUMATOID ARTHRITIS.—The temporomandibular joints frequently are involved in rheumatoid arthritis. The symptoms may be mild and go unnoticed, but if other joints are involved, the diagnosis is usually obvious. Occasionally the temporomandibular joint is the initial joint of complaint. In that case, the diagnosis may be difficult indeed.

Rheumatoid arthritis is an inflammatory condition of unknown etiology in which the inflamed and hypertrophic synovial membrane grows onto the articulating surfaces. The presence of such vascularized and innervated tissue on pressure-bearing surfaces of the joint causes pain and inflammation with normal functioning of the joint. It may also predispose to fibrous ankylosis. Rheumatoid arthritis is extremely variable in incidence, severity, and clinical course. Severe forms may cause bizarre resorption of the supporting osseous structures. Loss of vertical height due to condylar resorp-

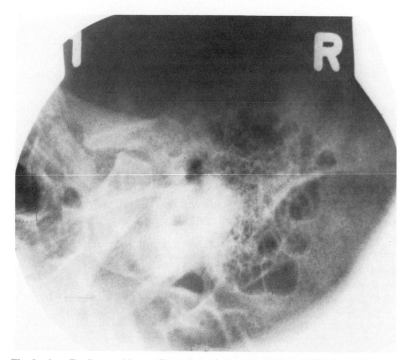

Fig 8–4.—Radiographic confirmation of degenerative arthritis in a 65-year-old woman. Transparietal projection of right temporomandibular joint in closed position. There is visible loss of contour of the subarticular osseous surfaces and irregularity of the width of the articular disc space. (From Bell W.E.: Temporomandibular joint, in Goldman H.M., Forrest S.P., Byrd D.L., et al. (eds.): *Current Therapy in Dentistry.* St. Louis, C.V. Mosby Co., 1968, vol. 3. Reproduced with permission.)

tion may induce a progressive open-bite relationship of the anterior teeth (see Fig 7–11). Diagnosis of rheumatoid arthritis requires medical confirmation.

HYPERURICEMIA.—An excessive level of serum uric acid causes a type of inflammatory arthritis in which pain with functional movements of the joint may be the chief complaint. This is also true of so-called subclinical gout, in which the serum uric acid level may run no higher than 6.0 mg/dl. As uric acid increases in concentration, the symptoms usually become greater. High levels may show deposits of urates in and about the joint. The symptoms are frequently polyarticular, episodic, and recurrent. It is seen more frequently in older persons. The diagnosis is confirmed by blood studies. The temporomandibular joints are involved with surprising frequency.

CHRONIC MANDIBULAR HYPOMOBILITIES

Another category of temporomandibular disorders has to do with *painless* restriction of mandibular movement. Such conditions may show signs of becoming progressively worse. When excessive force is used to move the mandible beyond the restraint imposed by such a condition, tethering adhesions may be injured and become inflamed, thus giving an element of pain to what otherwise is a painless disorder.

The clinical features that cause these conditions to be grouped together are

1. Restriction of mandibular movement
2. Painlessness (unless abused)
3. Chronicity

Depending on the location of the cause of restraint, these disorders are classified as (1) contracture of elevator muscles, (2) capsular fibrosis, and (3) ankylosis (Table 8–6). They are to be differentiated from the extra-articular restrictions of mandibular movement, described under the heading of *pseudoankylosis* (see chap. 7).

Contracture of Elevator Muscle(s)

Muscular contracture is regarded clinically as a reduction in the resting length of a muscle without seriously impairing its other functional capabilities. It is a painless condition unless injured by the application of forceful jaw opening, thus inducing myositis. Two types of muscle contracture are identifiable, namely, (1) *myostatic contracture,* which occurs as a result of failure to periodically stimulate the inverse stretch reflex, and (2) *myofibrotic contracture,* which occurs as a result of formation of excessive fibrous tissue within the muscle or its sheath. Myostatic contracture usually results from prolonged inability to open the mouth normally, the resting length of the elevator muscles decreasing until they conform to the degree of opening thus imposed. It may be reversible with proper therapy. Myofibrotic contracture is reactive to inflammation in and about the muscle and is not reversible.

The identifying characteristics of muscular contracture involving elevator masticatory muscles are:

1. History of prolonged myositic activity in the muscle or protracted restriction of mouth opening for any reason.
2. No pain, unless the muscles are injured by abusive efforts to open the mouth.
3. Restriction of mandibular movement, extracapsular in type, and involving opening movement only.

TABLE 8–6.—SYMPTOMS OF CHRONIC MANDIBULAR HYPOMOBILITIES

	CONTRACTURE OF ELEVATOR MUSCLE	CAPSULAR FIBROSIS	ANKYLOSIS
History	Prior protracted restriction of opening; Prior muscle trauma or inflammation	Prior trauma, surgery, or capsular inflammation	Prior trauma or infection
Masticatory pain	None, unless injured by excessive movement	None, unless injured by excessive movement	None, unless injured by excessive movement
Restriction of movement	Extracapsular restriction of condylar movement	Capsular restriction of condylar movement	Intracapsular restriction of condylar movement
Interference during movement	None	None	None
Acute malocclusion	None	None	None
Radiographic confirmation	Positive for extracapsular restraint of condyle	Positive for capsular restraint of condyle	Positive for intracapsular restraint of condyle

4. No interference during mandibular movements.

5. No acute malocclusion.

6. Radiographic confirmation of extracapsular restriction of mandibular movement, with condylar movement in open position being considerably less than in lateral position of the joint (see Fig 7–5).

Capsular Fibrosis (Contracture)

Fibrotic contracture of the capsular ligament is referred to as capsular fibrosis. It results from inflammation of the capsule, usually due to trauma. This includes surgery. The degree of restriction of mandibular movement depends on the resultant size of the capsule and thickness of the capsular wall. Capsular fibrosis restrains condylar movement in the outer ranges, imposing restriction on translatory movement of the condyle whether for opening, protrusion, or lateral excursion. It is painless unless force is used that causes injury to the capsule, thus inducing capsulitis. When this occurs, the true underlying condition may not become apparent until the acute symptoms subside. Then, evidence of preexisting capsular restriction of mandibular movement will remain.

The identifying characteristics of capsular fibrosis are:

1. History of prior trauma, surgery, or capsulitis.

2. No pain, unless the capsular ligament is abused by excessive translatory movements.

3. Capsular restriction of mandibular movement that restricts condylar movement in protrusion and lateral excursion to the same degree as in opening.

4. No interference during mandibular movement.

5. No acute malocclusion.

6. Radiographic confirmation of capsular restriction of mandibular movement, with condylar movement in open and lateral positions being identical and falling short of the crest of the articular eminence (see Fig 7–6).

Ankylosis

Intracapsular adhesions or actual ossification that tether condylar movement within the capsule is termed ankylosis. This results from trauma that causes hemarthrosis, which may organize and form a matrix for cicatrization. Although fibrous ankylosis is the usual type, occasionally ossification takes place (Fig 8–5). Ossification is more likely to occur when infection has been present. Ankylosis is usually unilateral because trauma is characteristically a single-joint affliction. It should be noted that when one joint is thus immobilized, degenerative change may take place in the opposite joint, due to the unnatural movements thus imposed.

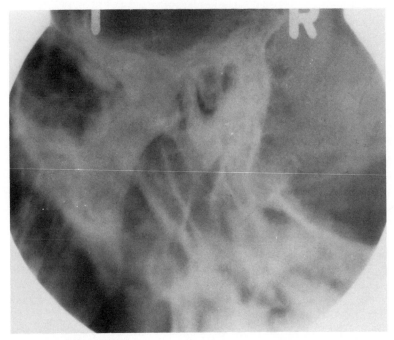

Fig 8–5.—Radiographic confirmation of osseous ankylosis in a 41-year-old man. Transparietal projection of right temporomandibular joint in closed position. The entire articular disc space is obscured by diffuse radiopaque deposition of dense osseous tissue.

Bilateral fibrous ankylosis may occur if the trauma is sufficient to cause hemarthrosis in both joints. This occurs with some frequency in small infants when the articular surfaces are still vascularized and vulnerable to injury that causes bleeding within the joints. A fall on the chin during the tottering stage may result in this condition. It may not be detected as a symptomatic disorder until many years later when restriction of opening and other movements are discovered, frequently as a result of dental treatment. Such patients chew vertically. When viewed in profile, they show no forward translation of the mandible with opening. Protrusive and lateral movements are nonexistent. Being a life-long condition, such abnormality in jaw function usually causes no subjective complaint because the individual has no knowledge of what normal mandibular movements are like. Only when strained by excessive opening or by forced lateral or protrusive movement—frequently by the dentist—does the condition become symptomatic. Pain results from injury to the tethering adhesions.

The degree to which fibrous ankylosis restricts jaw movement depends

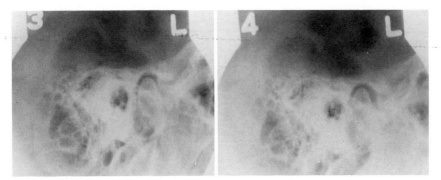

Fig 8–6.—Radiographic confirmation of fibrous ankylosis in a 16-year-old girl. Transparietal projection of left temporomandibular joint. *Left,* lateral excursion to the opposite side. *Right,* maximum opening. Condylar movement in lateral position is minimal. There is similar restriction of condylar movement in open position.

on the extent, location, and length of the fibrous adhesions. Tightly bound adhesions may restrict condylar movement to pure rotation, thus limiting comfortable opening to about 25 mm. The midline deflects ipsilaterally with both opening and protrusion. Longer and more flexible adhesions permit greater movement. The condition remains quite painless unless injured by excessive jaw movements.

Clinically, ankylosis should be differentiated from arrested mandibular movement due to protracted jamming of the articular disc and to protracted functional anterior dislocation of the disc. Ankylosis may be complicated by myostatic contracture of the elevator muscles due to protracted inability to open properly.

The identifying characteristics of ankylosis are:

1. History of prior injury or infection of the joint. The trauma may date back to a forceps delivery or an injury in early infancy.

2. No pain, unless the joint is abused.

3. Intracapsular restriction of mandibular movement.

4. No interference during mandibular movement.

5. No acute malocclusion.

6. Radiographic confirmation, with condylar restraint in open and lateral positions being identical and remaining fairly close to the closed-joint position (Fig 8–6).

GROWTH DISORDERS OF THE JOINT

Disorders of growth that afflict the craniomandibular articulation are varied. Fortunately, growth disorders that are of sufficient importance to become symptomatic are low in incidence. They have several features that are similar enough to justify grouping them together, namely:

1. The clinical symptoms occur directly from the structural changes that are present.

2. Disturbance in function and the incidence of masticatory pain are secondary to those structural changes.

3. Radiographic evidence is of primary importance in differential diagnosis.

For sake of discussion, disorders of growth may be divided into three categories, namely, (1) aberrations related to the developmental process, (2) acquired changes in structural form, and (3) neoplasia. For more adequate discussion of disorders of this type, authoritative sources of information are available.[3, 7-9]

Aberration of Development

A wide variation in size and shape of temporomandibular joint structure can be considered within normal limits. Even when structural variation exceeds what usually is considered normal, masticatory function may remain nonsymptomatic. It is when deficiency, hyperplasia, or asymmetry imposes a measure of dysfunction on the masticatory apparatus that symptoms become apparent. The cause of such aberration of development is either unknown or poorly understood. Deficiency problems are usually bilateral and symmetric. Some are associated with facial defects.

Bilateral hyperplasia results in mandibular prognathism; unilateral overgrowth causes facial asymmetry. When these conditions develop from an early age, quite satisfactory compensatory adjustment of the joints and den-

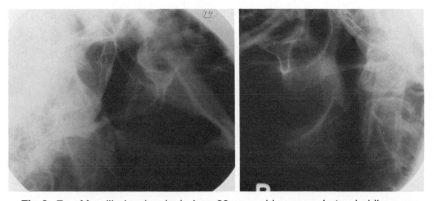

Fig 8-7.—Mandibular dysplasia in a 60-year-old woman. Lateral oblique projection of left and right mandibular rami. Note that structural formation of the right side is normal. Left side shows agenesis of entire condylar process and most of the mandibular ramus.

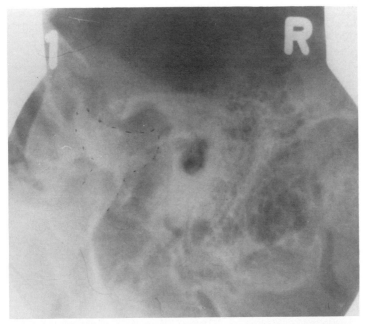

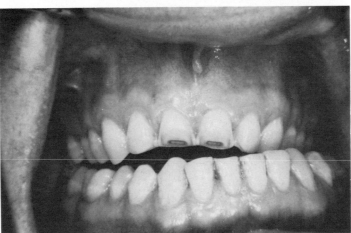

Fig 8–8.—Radiographic confirmation of aberration of growth of the mandibular condyle in a 30-year-old man. *Top,* transparietal projection of right temporomandibular joint in closed position. Note the shape of condyle, with enlargement posteriorly as well as anteriorly. The posterior enlargement has shifted the position of the condyle anteriorly, thus causing gross malocclusion. *Bottom,* dentition occludes in cross-bite to the left side. (From Bell W.E.: Management of temporomandibular joint problems, in Goldman H.M., Gilmore H.W., Royer R.Q., et al. (eds.): *Current Therapy in Dentistry.* St. Louis, C.V. Mosby Co., 1970, vol. 4. Reproduced with permission.)

tition may take place, so that very little, if any, functional incompatibility (occlusal disharmony) is evident, even though improper articulation of the teeth may be obvious.

Dysplasia of the mandible as well as of the temporal bone is usually unilateral and asymmetric. Although the cause of such condition is not known precisely, experimental evidence indicates that a hematoma during the critical developmental period can cause similar defects.[7] Complete agenesis of the condyle may occur (Fig 8–7).

Acquired Change in Joint Structure

Some anomalies of growth occur after joint development and dentition are complete. Unilateral hyperplasia of the condyloid process in adults may cause marked malocclusion, such as cross-bite, thus creating structural incompatibility of the parts (Fig 8–8).

Perhaps the most frequently acquired change in joint structure occurs as a result of trauma. Actual alteration in the osseous relationship may result

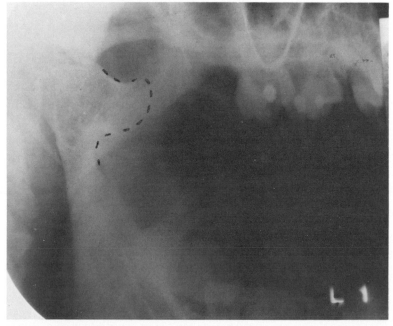

Fig 8–9.—Radiographic confirmation of aberration of condylar growth due to benign neoplasia in a 41-year-old man. Transfacial projection of left mandibular condyle shows marked enlargement of the osseous structure anteriorly. Note that the superior surface of new growth conforms in shape to the fossa and articular eminence, evidence of slow, benign growth.

from fracture of the condyloid process. Traumatized bone may react by developing hypertrophic outgrowths that can become incompatible with normal joint function (see Fig 8–3).

Ordinarily, all such aberrations of growth remain nonsymptomatic until the structural change interferes with normal functioning of the joint and/or dentition. The final symptomatology, therefore, is varied and depends on the particular situation at hand.

Neoplasia

Neoplastic involvement of a temporomandibular joint is relatively rare. Tumors of cartilage and osseous structure are reported most frequently. Osteoma of the condyle may be extremely difficult to distinguish from hyperplasia. Chondroma, osteochondroma, giant cell granuloma, and hemangioma have been reported. All such tumors involving the mandibular condyle are extremely rare (Fig 8–9).

Although primary malignant disease of the temporomandibular joint proper has been reported, direct invasion from surrounding structures is considerably more frequent. When this occurs, the initial joint complaint is usually painless restriction of joint movement, which is highly suggestive of fibrous ankylosis. It is only when the disorder expresses itself as a progressively worsening condition with an increasing component of pain that malignancy may be suspected (Fig 8–10). Needle biopsy can help make a positive diagnosis.

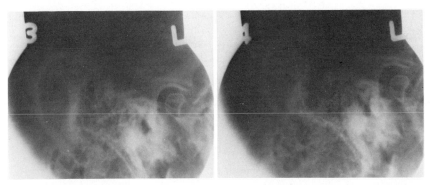

Fig 8–10.—Radiographic confirmation of fixation of the temporomandibular joint due to extra-articular cause, later determined to be invasion by malignant neoplasm, in a 54-year-old woman. Transparietal projection of the left temporomandibular joint. *Left,* lateral excursion to the opposite side; *right,* maximum opening. Note that there is marked restriction of mandibular movement in both lateral excursion and opening, but not to exactly the same degree. The movement with opening slightly exceeds that of lateral excursion, a finding that is inconsistent with intracapsular restraint of mandibular movement.

REFERENCES

1. Bell W.E.: Clinical diagnosis of the pain-dysfunction syndrome. *J. Am. Dent. Assoc.* 79:154, 1969.
2. Bell W.E.: *Orofacial Pains, Differential Diagnosis*, ed. 2. Chicago, Year Book Medical Publishers, 1979.
3. Cherrick H.M.: Pathology, in Sarnat B.G., Laskin D.M. (eds.): *The Temporomandibular Joint*, ed. 3. Springfield, Ill., Charles C Thomas, Publisher, 1979, pp. 180–204.
4. Greene C.S.: Myofascial pain-dysfunction syndrome: The evolution of concepts, in Sarnat B.G., Laskin D.M. (eds.): *The Temporomandibular Joint*, ed. 3. Springfield, Ill., Charles C Thomas, Publisher, 1979, pp. 277–288.
5. Klinenberg J.R.: The arthritides, in Sarnat B.G., Laskin D.M. (eds.): *The Temporomandibular Joint*, ed. 3. Springfield, Ill., Charles C Thomas, Publisher, 1979, pp. 335–347.
6. Laskin D.M.: Etiology of the pain-dysfunction syndrome. *J. Am. Dent. Assoc.* 79:147, 1969.
7. Poswillo D.E.: Congenital malformations: Prenatal experimental studies, in Sarnat B.G., Laskin D.M. (eds.): *The Temporomandibular Joint*, ed. 3. Springfield, Ill., Charles C Thomas, Publisher, 1979, pp. 127–150.
8. Ross R.B.: Developmental anomalies and dysfunctions of the temporomandibular joint, in Zarb G.A., Carlsson G.E. (eds.): *Temporomandibular Joint Function and Dysfunction*. Copenhagen, Munksgaard, 1979, pp. 119–154.
9. Sarnat B.G., Laskin D.M.: Surgical considerations, in Sarnat B.G., Laskin D.M. (eds.): *The Temporomandibular Joint*, ed. 3. Springfield, Ill., Charles C Thomas, Publisher, 1979, pp. 433–470.
10. Schwartz L.L.: A temporomandibular joint pain-dysfunction syndrome. *J. Chron. Dis.* 3:284, 1956.
11. Wolff H.G.: *Headache and Other Head Pain*, ed. 2. New York, Oxford University Press, 1963, p. 606.

9 / Collection and Evaluation of Diagnostic Data

THE MANAGEMENT of temporomandibular disorders requires adequate and accurate information concerning:

1. The functional anatomy of the craniomandibular articulation and masticatory musculature.

2. Principles of biomechanics as they apply to functioning of the articular disc.

3. Principles of muscle physiology as they apply to movements of the mandible and the articular disc.

4. Standards of normal by which masticatory function can be judged.

5. An understanding of pain in general and masticatory pains in particular.

6. Criteria for identifying various masticatory symptoms.

7. Full awareness of the gamut of disorders that afflict the masticatory apparatus.

Proper programming of the dentist's CNS computer requires a great deal of information on all these levels. A deficiency at any point may have decisive effect on the end results.

Assuming that all essential information has been acquired, effective management begins with making an accurate diagnosis. This falls into two parts, namely, the collection of diagnostic data and the proper evaluation of that data. The collection of data (making an examination) is largely a technical procedure, much of which can be accomplished by nonprofessional technicians. It is the evaluation of the data (making a diagnosis) that requires the programming mentioned above.

COLLECTION OF DIAGNOSTIC DATA

To initiate an examination of the craniomandibular articulation and masticatory musculature, one first should identify the patient's complaint.

Chief Complaint

The patient's complaint should be recorded in his own language, for this is going to be the final issue upon which he will judge the effectiveness of your management of his problem. It is important to keep in mind that this is *his complaint,* and what is chief to him is what it is all about.

Then, the complaint should be restated in the technical language of masticatory symptomatology as reviewed in chapters 6 and 7. This statement of the problem should be the primary issue when evaluation of the data is made and a diagnosis rendered. This should be the primary condition for which treatment is planned.

Identification of Masticatory Symptoms

The next step in data collection is the clear identification of all masticatory and concomitant symptoms, noting how they relate to the chief complaint and to each other. These should be divided into clinically recognizable conditions of (1) pain, (2) restriction of mandibular movement, (3) interference during mandibular movement, (4) acute malocclusion, and (5) concomitant symptoms.

MASTICATORY PAIN.—Any complaint of pain should be classified according to its clinical characteristics as musculoskeletal pain of the deep somatic category.[1] Its true site of origin should be located clinically by manual palpation and functional manipulation. If possible, secondary pains due to central excitatory effects at least should be suspected. A general classification of myalgia or arthralgia should be made.

RESTRICTION OF JAW MOVEMENT.—Any restriction of jaw movement should be noted in either joint as related to opening, protrusion, and lateral excursion. Bilateral symmetry of movement should be checked. Restrictions that appear to relate to the inhibitory effects of pain rather than to structural causes should be noted. Deflections of the midline incisal path with opening and protrusion should be graphed. A clinical impression of whether the restriction is extra-articular (pseudoankylosis) or articular should be made. If articular, it should be classified as extracapsular, capsular, or intracapsular in location.

INTERFERENCE DURING JAW MOVEMENTS.—Abnormal sensations, noises, and movements during translatory cycles induced by opening-closing, protrusion-retrusion, and lateral excursion and return (in both pivoting and translating joints) should be identified. Such symptoms should be classified as to how they relate to the translatory cycle. Deviations of the midline incisal path during opening-closing should be graphed. The effect of power strokes (using chewing gum or peanuts) and maximum intercuspation should be noted, as they relate to the various chewing movements on both the biting and the nonbiting sides.

ACUTE MALOCCLUSION.—Malocclusion of which the patient is fully aware and which constitutes at least a part of his complaint should be identified. Any such acute malocclusion should be described in terms of overstressed or understressed teeth, premature striking or disocclusion of teeth, cross-bite, or open-bite.

Concomitant Symptoms

Related orofacial, head, and cervical pains should be noted and described. Their clinical characteristics should be recorded to help identify the proper category and type of pain they represent. The true source of such pain should be determined and secondary central excitatory effects identified, if possible. Ear symptoms should be described. Note should be taken of any obvious deviation in the postural relationship between the mandible and the cervical structures.

Etiologic Considerations

Obtaining an adequate history is essential because in it usually may be found the best clues to possible etiology. The history should be divided into three parts, namely, (1) general personal physical history of the patient as it relates to the present complaint, (2) specific historical information related to the initiation of the complaint, and (3) a past chronological record of the behavior of each of the masticatory symptoms identified above, especially as they relate to each other.

GENERAL PERSONAL HISTORY.—Consideration should be given to anomalous development, acquired aberrations of growth, previous (even childhood) injuries, illnesses, joint complaints, muscle complaints, and emotional disturbances. The masticatory history should include chewing problems, malocclusion, abusive habits, and mannerisms; bruxism; dentition problems; and extensive dental, orthodontic, or surgical treatment involving the masticatory apparatus. Previous symptoms or similar episodes should be recorded.

SPECIFIC HISTORY RELATIVE TO THE COMPLAINT.—Note should be taken of any prior illness, physical fatigue, emotional crisis, injury, episode of pain about the head or neck, dental treatment, local or general anesthesia, or any alteration in the way the teeth, mouth, and jaws have been used. Any feeling of change in the bite; sensation of fatigue or muscle weakness in the jaws; or feeling of prior stiffness, catching, joint noise, or other unusual sensation should be recorded. Insomnia, restlessness, early morning fatigue, known increase in bruxism, or sensation of overstressed teeth should be taken into account. Questions that tend to reveal the presence of unusually high emotional tension should be asked. All medications currently being used, and what they are prescribed for, should be reviewed. Such information may be obtained from the patient's physician, if the exact content of medications is not known.

CHRONOLOGICAL RECORD OF SYMPTOM BEHAVIOR.—Each masticatory symptom, as identified above, should be traced chronologically from its inception to the present. It should be noted how they relate to each other in timing and how they relate to function, temporal patterns, known aggravating factors, and therapeutic efforts.

Functional Manipulations

The next step in the collection of data is to determine how the masticatory symptoms react under the impact of provocative or ameliorating functional manipulations. *It is important that the effect of power strokes be analyzed as well as empty-mouth movements.* Several maneuvers are useful in obtaining this information, as noted below.

SWALLOWING AND TONGUE MOVEMENTS.—Pain should be examined as it relates to tongue and throat movements by stabilizing the mandible with a small mouth prop. Note should be taken of how the symptoms relate to the swallowing of saliva, fluids, and solid foods.

CLINICAL IDENTIFICATION OF GROSS OCCLUSAL DISHARMONY.—By lightly "tap-tapping" the teeth together in the relaxed closed relationship of the joint, gross occlusal disharmony may be sensed as lack of simultaneous contact of the teeth. Clenching the teeth may identify disoccluded or overstressed teeth. When the teeth are firmly occluded from the unclenched closed position *without separating the teeth,* gross movement between the teeth may be identified, either sensed subjectively by the patient or felt with the examiner's fingers placed along the occluded teeth. Gross lateral displacement may be seen as movement at the midline of the incisors.

EFFECT OF MAXIMUM INTERCUSPATION.—Clenching the teeth from the relaxed closed (unclenched) position yields the effect of maximum intercuspation. This should be done with and without any dental appliances that are normally used. It should be noted if symptoms relate to the act of clenching or occur as biting stress is released. Any alteration of symptoms due to biting against a thin separator placed ipsilaterally, contralaterally, or bilaterally between the teeth should be observed. Any alteration of symptoms due to biting against a thick separator or biting in a slightly protruded relationship should be noted.

OPENING-CLOSING MOVEMENTS.—The interincisal distance of maximum opening should be measured. The total opening should be recorded as this interincisal distance *plus the overbite* when the teeth are occluded. If opening displays deflection of the midline, the *straight-line opening* should be measured also. If deviation of the midline takes place, any alteration in symptoms due to faster opening movement should be noted. Opening against resistance should be done. *The effect of power strokes should be observed.* A comparison should be made of any difference in symptoms as a result of opening from a firmly occluded position or from a relaxed resting position. Note should be taken of symptoms that relate to power strokes that end in maximum intercuspation, in contrast to a resting or separated position.

PROTRUSION-RETRUSION MOVEMENTS.—Maximum protrusion should be measured. Such measurement should take into account any overjet that is present when the teeth are occluded. If the midline deflects, then the guided straight-line protrusion should be measured also. Special note should be taken of the extent of deflection of the midline. Protrusion against resistance should be attempted. Note should be taken of symptoms due to a power stroke. This should be done on both the biting and the nonbiting sides.

LATERAL MOVEMENT TO THE OPPOSITE SIDE.—Maximum lateral movements should be measured and compared for symmetry. If considerable effort is required to make such movements, the unstrained movements should be measured also. Note should be taken of difference in symptoms in the pivoting and the balancing joint. Lateral movement against resistance should be attempted. Any irregularity in jaw movement observed during lateral excursions, or the return movements, should be noted. Note should be taken of symptoms due to excursions and power returns.

CLINICAL EVALUATION OF DATA

The data gleaned from the chief complaint, the masticatory and concomitant symptoms, the case history, and the functional manipulations of the joints should be summarized carefully and put into usable form. This is done best by arranging the summarized data into a standard sequence, as follows:

1. Features in the history that are etiologically significant.
2. Data relating to symptoms of masticatory pain, including (1) the identifying clinical characteristics that place the complaint into the deep, musculoskeletal category, and (2) clinical characteristics that identify the pain as either myogenous, arthralgic, or both.
3. Data relating to the restriction of mandibular movement, including

whether the location of such restriction is extracapsular, capsular, or intra-capsular.

4. Data relating to symptoms of interference during mandibular move-ments (abnormal sensations, noises, and/or movements), including (1) the classification of such interference as it relates to the translatory cycle, (2) whether it appears to relate to excessive passive interarticular pressure, lack of compatibility of the sliding surfaces, or impaired disc-condyle com-plex function (if such disorder is of the Class III category), (3) whether it identifies arrested movement between the articular disc and condyle, dam-age to the articular disc proper, dysfunctional discal ligaments, or dysfunc-tional superior retrodiscal lamina (if impaired disc-condyle complex func-tioning is evident), and (4) whether it identifies general disc mal-functioning, functional displacement of the disc, or functional dislocation of the articular disc (if such interference relates to impaired discal ligaments).

5. Data relating to identifiable acute malocclusion, including whether it appears to be muscle-induced or joint-induced.

With the summarized data thus arranged, it is much easier to make the necessary comparisons that effectuate a tentative clinical diagnosis.

Tentative Clinical Diagnosis

The development of a clinical diagnosis can be taken in steps. With the summarized data at hand, comparison first should be made with the stan-dards of normal (see chap. 5). Second, those data that clearly depart from normal should be listed according to the type of symptom, namely, pain, restriction of mandibular movement, interference during mandibular movement, and acute malocclusion. Each should be evaluated in terms of definite clinical criteria (see chaps. 6 and 7). The third step is to compare these symptomatic criteria with the gamut of classified temporomandibular disorders (see chap. 8 and Table 8–1).

A decision then should be made as to whether the tentative clinical di-agnosis has sufficient merit and reasonableness to warrant initiating man-agement procedures or whether further confirmation is needed. Ordinar-ily, if palliative therapy is expected to effectively manage the complaint, further confirmation, other than therapeutic trial, may be superfluous. But, if any question remains, and especially if definitive therapy includes non-reversible dental or joint treatment measures, positive confirmation should be obtained.

CONFIRMATION OF CLINICAL DIAGNOSIS

Confirmation of the clinical diagnosis can be accomplished by employing one or more of several diagnostic procedures, namely, (1) analgesic blocking to confirm the source of pain, (2) radiography, (3) laboratory studies, (4) consultation with other professionals, and (5) clinical trial therapy.

Analgesic Blocking

When positive confirmation of the true source of pain is needed, especially when it is necessary to distinguish between primary pain and referred pain or secondary hyperalgesia, skillful use of local anesthesia is dependable and accurate.[1] The following general rules should be followed:

1. Actively inflamed structures should be avoided.

2. Acceptable aseptic technique should be followed routinely.

3. One should be thoroughly familiar with all anatomical structures through which the needle is to pass.

4. One should be thoroughly familiar with the solution to be used, especially its proper dosage, contraindications, and possible side effects.

5. Invariably, one should aspirate prior to injecting the solution.

It should be noted that good local anesthesia of skeletal muscle tissue requires that the solution contain no epinephrine-like substance. Also, muscle tissue usually requires somewhat more time for anesthesia to become effective (5 minutes or more).

As a general rule, muscle injections are preferred to those for anesthesia of the joint proper. To obtain satisfactory anesthesia of the joint, two injections are needed: (1) an infiltration of solution at a point just posterior to the neck of the condyloid process to anesthetize the auriculotemporal nerve and (2) a small infiltration just anterior to the joint proper to anesthetize the anterior third of the capsular ligament.

The local anesthetic injections for the main masticatory muscles by the extraoral route are illustrated in Figures 9–1 through 9–4. It should be understood that injections about the temporomandibular area may include motor fibers of the facial nerve. This may induce paralysis of the eyelid for the duration of anesthesia. Patients should be forewarned.

Every practitioner who is serious about temporomandibular disorders should make himself especially proficient in the use of local analgesic blocking techniques. When needed, there is no substitute. This method is extremely useful both diagnostically and therapeutically. The minor injury such injections may cause is more than justified by the benefit obtained.

Radiography

Radiographic visualization has essential confirming value. The tissue injury induced by radiation is usually justified by the information gained. *It should not be used as a substitute for clinical diagnosis; it has too many limitations.* But its confirming value is great indeed. Practitioners who are

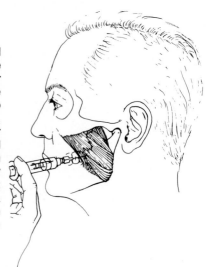

Fig 9–1.—Technique for external injection of masseter muscle. The needle enters the muscle at the anterior border about midbody and is passed through the muscle at several angles and depths to reach the deep and superficial layers. With each pass of the needle, after aspirating it, the solution is deposited slowly as the needle is withdrawn. (From Bell W.E.: Management of masticatory pain, in Alling C.C., Mahan P.E. (eds.): *Facial Pain,* ed. 2. Philadelphia, Lea & Febiger, 1977. Reproduced with permission.)

serious about complaints of the masticatory system should become proficient in temporomandibular radiographic technique. This is something that cannot be delegated to a technician or specialist, because much of its value depends on precise control of the joint positions viewed—something best done by the examiner himself.

Radiographic methods may be classified into several technical groups, namely

1. Ordinary transcranial projection
2. Panoramic projection

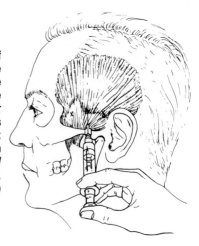

Fig 9–2.—Technique for injection of temporalis muscle. Needle penetrates the muscle at several points *(X)* just above the zygomatic arch to reach most of the fibers. With each penetration, after aspirating the needle, solution is deposited slowly. (From Bell W.E.: Management of masticatory pain, in Alling C.C., Mahan P.E. (eds.): *Facial Pain,* ed. 2. Philadelphia, Lea & Febiger, 1977. Reproduced with permission.)

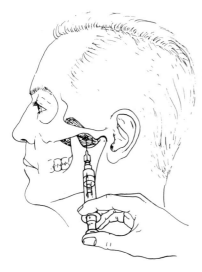

Fig 9–3.—Technique for external injection of lateral pterygoid muscle. After the needle is passed through the mandibular sigmoid notch, it is directed slightly upward and inward to a total depth of 35 to 40 mm. After aspiration of the needle, the solution is deposited slowly. Motor fibers of the facial nerve also may be anesthetized. (From Bell W.E.: Management of masticatory pain, in Alling C.C., Mahan P.E. (eds.): *Facial Pain*, ed. 2. Philadelphia, Lea & Febiger, 1977. Reproduced with permission.)

3. Tomographic projection
4. Fluoroscopy
5. Cinefluoroscopy

Arthrography is accomplished by injecting a radiopaque contrast medium into the joint cavity (or cavities) to render the synovial fluid radiopaque. It can be adapted to any of the above techniques but has its greatest value when applied to the tomographic and cinefluoroscopic methods. Although temporomandibular arthrography has been used for many years,[4] it has recently become popular as the importance of internal derangements of the

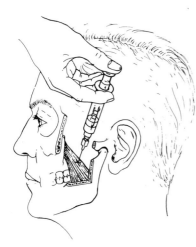

Fig 9–4.—Technique for external injection of medial pterygoid muscle. After the needle is passed through the mandibular sigmoid notch, it is directed boldly downward and inward to a total depth of about 40 mm. After aspiration of the needle, the solution is deposited slowly. Motor fibers of the facial nerve also may be anesthetized. (From Bell W.E.: Management of masticatory pain, in Alling C.C., Mahan P.E. (eds.): *Facial Pain*, ed. 2. Philadelphia, Lea & Febiger, 1977. Reproduced with permission.)

joint has become better understood.[2, 3, 6] It has positive value in detecting perforations in the articular disc that permit exchange of synovial fluid between the two cavities.[5] The clinical significance of such defect, however, has not been established. This method gives information on the thickness of radiolucent tissue on the subarticular osseous structures (condyle and temporal articular facet) and helps to visualize displacement of the articular disc from the mandibular condyle. Presently, the effect of a radiopaque *hypertonic solution* on normal disc function is not known. The configuration of *distended* synovial cavities as seen in "normal" joint arthrography may or may not represent the true conditions that prevail. Although it appears that considerable reliance can be placed on the shape of the radiopaque material within the joint as being indicative of disc position, it is suggested that the radiographic appearance be used to *confirm the clinical criteria* by which such abnormalities can be identified, rather than as the primary positive diagnostic procedure. This word of caution is not intended to discourage the use of arthrography. Rather, it is intended to point up the limitations of all forms of radiography in temporomandibular diagnosis. *The greatest value of radiography in the management of temporomandibular disorders is to confirm clinical evidence.*

ORDINARY TRANSCRANIAL PROJECTION.—This method has limitations that should be fully understood and appreciated. It does not visualize the true subarticular osseous surfaces, but rather the outer lateral margins of the joint. Thus, the true articular disc space is not seen. If critical evaluation of the articular disc space or the subarticular osseous structures is needed, the tomographic method in the upright sitting position is required. Information concerning articular disc behavior must be *inferred from changes in width and position* of the so-called joint-gap space in the condyle-disc-eminence relationship as viewed in different functional positions of the joint. Although this method involves considerable radiation, it does have the striking advantage of *availability*. The technique is easy and can be accomplished with ordinary dental x-ray equipment.

This method yields a great deal of information in spite of its limitations. Fairly accurate estimate of the inclination of the articular eminence is available by comparing with the shadow of the supra-articular crest in the region of the eminence, the crest being nearly parallel to the Frankfurt plane. The shape and gross structure of the subarticular bone is visualized. Films of the joints should be done in series so as to give information about joint functioning. Such a series should include at least four joint positions, namely, (1) closed unclenched position, (2) closed clenched position, (3) maximum unstrained lateral position (excursion to the opposite side), and (4) maximum unstrained open position. By comparing such radiographs with the known radiographic standards of normal (see chap. 5), departures from normal joint structure and function become obvious (see Fig 5–3).

The transcranial projections can be supplemented with a transpharyngeal (transfacial) projection to visualize the mandibular condyle in profile and with transorbital projections to visualize the condyle frontally.

PANORAMIC PROJECTION.—Panoramic projection of the facial bones, including the temporomandibular joints, provides a useful screening visualization of the masticatory structures. Since it is done in a single static position, its value is seriously limited. It often furnishes clues that justify more adequate radiographic examination of the joints.

TOMOGRAPHIC PROJECTION.—Tomography affords the most accurate radiographic visualization of the temporomandibular joint. If the patient is positioned in the upright sitting posture, films made by this method *in properly controlled series* are an excellent means of measuring accurately the articular disc space during functional movements of the joint. This offers a good chance of radiographically discerning abnormalities of articular disc function, even though the disc itself is not visible.

FLUOROSCOPY.—Fluoroscopy offers the marked advantage of visualizing movement of the bony parts. However, it embodies all the limitations of the ordinary transcranial projection.

CINEFLUOROSCOPY.—Although this method retains the limitations of flat-plate radiography, it provides a graphic record that permits frame-by-frame study, review, comparison, and measurement. Thus, joint movements under controlled functional conditions can be recorded and scrutinized. Both sagittal and frontal viewing can be done.

Regardless of the method used and whether a contrast medium is injected, one caution should be sounded concerning radiographic interpretation of temporomandibular joint functioning. By observing only the condyle and articular eminence with an intervening space, the temptation is great to think of the condyle as articulating with that eminence, the space between representing a "meniscus" separating the two bony parts. It is important to keep in mind that the condyle articulates rather with an invisible articular disc, thus forming a hinge-like disc-condyle complex. It is this invisible complex that articulates with the articular eminence as a sliding joint. *Unless the examiner disciplines himself always to keep these facts in mind, the gross movements that are so graphically demonstrated may be misleading indeed.*

Laboratory Studies

Several laboratory tests may help confirm specific disorders of the temporomandibular joints. The serum uric acid test is essential to the diagnosis of hyperuricemia. Sedimentation rate and latex fixation test, a serologic test for rheumatoid factor, are useful in making a diagnosis of rheumatoid arthritis. Negative findings, however, do not preclude the disease. Synovial fluid examination and blood studies may be needed to confirm synovitis and infectious inflammatory arthritis.

Consultations

Some conditions may require the opinion of other practitioners, both dental and medical. Dental specialists may be needed to help settle questions about occlusion, oral rehabilitation, and surgical considerations. Medical specialists that may help resolve certain questions include otolaryngologists, neurologists, orthopedists, anesthesiologists, internists, psychologists, and physiotherapists.

Clinical Trial

Response to therapy is not to be ignored for its confirming value. To attest the correctness of a diagnosis, one should be familiar with placebo effect, which accounts for up to about 35% to 40% of the effectiveness of any treatment. If benefit from initial therapy well exceeds placebo effect, it is presumptive evidence that the diagnosis is correct and the treatment proper.

It is wise, however, to use only reversible palliative therapy for its confirming value. All serious definitive and especially irreversible therapy should await a confirmed working diagnosis.

FINAL EVALUATION OF DATA

A confirmed working diagnosis should be the objective of every examination. When all the clinical data are collected and evaluated and a tentative clinical diagnosis has been made, a serious attempt should be made to confirm the diagnosis by one or more of the several means discussed, if no more than by trial therapy. Only when positive confirmation is established can one really plan and embark on definitive therapy with predictive effectiveness.

It should be the rule to judge the effectiveness of therapy on a continuing basis. At any time that serious inconsistency in the management of a temporomandibular disorder becomes evident, it is well to suspend further treatment until such is reasonably resolved. *Relapse soon after treatment, recurrence or persistence of symptoms, and chronicity without organic justification are warning signals that should be heeded.* Caution should always be exercised, especially when irreversible therapeutic measures are undertaken.

REFERENCES

1. Bell W.E.: *Orofacial Pains, Differential Diagnosis,* ed. 2. Chicago, Year Book Medical Publishers, 1979.
2. Blaschke D.D., Solberg W.K., Sanders B.: Arthrography of the temporomandibular joint: Review of current status, *J. Am. Dent. Assoc.* 100:388, 1980.
3. Farrar W.B., McCarty W.L.: Inferior joint space arthrography and characteristics of condylar paths in internal derangements of the TMJ. *J. Pros. Dent.* 41:548, 1979.
4. Norgaard F.: *Temporomandibular Arthrography.* Copenhagen, Munksgaard, 1947.
5. Oberg T.: Radiology of the temporomandibular joint, in Solberg W.K., Clark G.T. (eds.): *Temporomandibular Joint Problems.* Chicago, Quintessence Publishing Co., 1980, pp. 49–68.
6. Wilkes C.H.: Arthrography of the temporomandibular joint in patients with the TMJ pain-dysfunction syndrome. *Minn. Med.* 61:645, 1978.

10 / Guidelines for the Treatment of Temporomandibular Disorders

THE MOST IMPORTANT INITIAL STEP in therapy is an accurate diagnosis. Nothing can take its place. *Diagnosis always precedes treatment.* Assuming that a diagnosis has been made, including what is wrong, where, and why, one should be able to make a reasonably accurate prognosis as to how the future will unfold. One should be able to predict to what degree therapy can be expected to produce favorable results, something of the time factor involved, what treatment modalities may be required, and what residual or progressive symptoms or conditions may remain for future consideration.

PALLIATIVE TREATMENT

Palliative therapy includes measures that can be taken to give the patient some comfort while more serious efforts are under way to find out the facts in the case and plan more definitive treatment. In temporomandibular disorders, two forms of therapy are indicated, regardless of what the final state of affairs may be, namely, reduction of pain and restriction of functional demands.

Control of Pain

It is important that pain be controlled with dispatch. But one should not underestimate the value of pain as a diagnostic symptom, as a deterrent to restrain abusive joint use, and as a means of judging progress in the resolution of a complaint. Certainly no effort should be made to eliminate pain entirely, and the patient should be so informed. If pain is eliminated completely, the patient loses his number-one signal to stop doing whatever it is that hurts.

Analgesic medications may be needed. If the patient is persuaded to restrict jaw use within painless limits, enough benefit usually accrues that simple household pain remedies may suffice. Narcotic analgesics should be avoided as much as possible because of their undesirable effects: nausea, constipation, respiratory depression, hypotension, and possible dependence. They should be used with caution, preferably under active medical supervision, in patients with head injuries, patients suffering from asthma, patients recently treated with monoamine oxidase inhibitors, and patients that are pregnant or nursing. All analgesics should be restricted to dosage that will make the pain tolerable without eliminating it completely.

Other useful palliative measures are available for the control of pain, such as (1) stimulation of superficial cutaneous receptors by light massage, thermal applications, hydrotherapy, vapocoolants, vibration, electroanalgesia, and transcutaneous nerve stimulators, and (2) suggestion, distraction, and good rapport.

Restriction of Functional Demands

Chewing and all jaw use should be restricted voluntarily within painless limits. This means alteration of the diet and modification of chewing habits. Foods should be softer, bites smaller, chewing movements slower. Clenching the teeth should be avoided.

DEFINITIVE THERAPY

In all planning for the definitive correction of temporomandibular complaints, the patient should be brought actively into the program so that he may assume his burden of responsibility for the effectiveness of therapy. Being musculoskeletal in type, all such complaints of the masticatory system have an interlocking relationship with masticatory function. This is where the patient comes into the problem: *he is the source and determinant of function.* He cannot avoid sharing responsibility for the effectiveness of therapy, and he must know this.

As a general rule, therapy consists of (1) elimination of the cause(s) and (2) resolution of the symptoms and care of the damaged parts.

Elimination of the Cause

The first step in definitive treatment is to eliminate or neutralize the cause of the condition. This may apply to predisposing factors and activating factors.

PREDISPOSING FACTORS.—Chronic occlusal disharmony may be a predisposing factor in many temporomandibular disorders. Slight disharmony may initiate sensory and proprioceptive input that is answered by acute muscle disorders. More severe disharmony that causes gross displacement of the disc-condyle complex during maximum intercuspation predisposes to interference disorders of the joint. Such destructive changes may involve the osseous-supported articular surfaces, the articular discs, the structures of the disc-condyle complex (especially the discal ligaments), the temporomandibular ligament, and the retrodiscal tissue. Elimination of such chronic occlusal disharmony is mandatory. The timing of correction, however, may vary, depending on the type of disorder present and whether a component of acute malocclusion is to be taken into account.

Skeletal and craniofacial disharmony as well as former trauma to the facial structures are important factors that influence functioning of the masticatory apparatus, particularly the disc-condyle complex. The elimination of such causes is not a practical consideration. Rather, it should be an objective of therapy to minimize, if not eliminate entirely, the effects of such factors.

Very important predisposing factors are abnormal or excessive functional demands, such as habitual excessive use of chewing force, abusive mannerisms, using the teeth and jaws for nonmasticatory purposes, and bruxism. Usually, habit training can be successfully employed to minimize such conditions, including bruxism, which no doubt is the most difficult of all to manage. Daytime bruxism may be controlled by habit training to voluntarily leave the teeth separated or ajar. The use of reminders, such as a small piece of chewing gum patted along the occlusal surfaces of the molar teeth, may be helpful. Nighttime bruxism may be reduced by sleeping flat on the back without a pillow, by autosuggestion that "I will not clench my teeth while asleep!," or by positive posthypnotic suggestion. Sometimes, a nightguard device that separates the teeth helps to control the condition.

ACTIVATING FACTORS.—The most important activating cause of temporomandibular disorders is emotional tension. It is a major cause of bruxism, of excessive passive interarticular pressure, and of many acute muscle disorders. Tension control programs may include (1) medicinal therapy in the form of tranquilizers and muscle relaxants; (2) psychological care in the form of counseling, autosuggestion, hypnotherapy, or psychotherapy; (3) biofeedback techniques; and (4) genuine understanding and empathy by which the burden of being human is made more tolerable.

An important activator of acute muscle spasm is the continuous input of deep-pain impulses that initiate central excitatory effects. To eliminate this important and frequent cause requires the skillful identification and eradication of the primary pain source—which may not be related to the masticatory system, or even to dentistry. Very careful differential diagnosis of orofacial pain syndromes is prerequisite to success.[4]

Resolution of Symptoms and Care of Damaged Parts

Structural changes in the musculature and joints do not go away simply because etiologic factors are eliminated. Natural resolution may occur, is always desirable, and should be taken into consideration in treatment planning. Indeed, the temporomandibular joints are constructed favorably for this, in that the articular surfaces are fibrous tissue rather than cartilaginous. As a rule, however, special measures are required for damaged parts to be brought within the limit of tolerability for the patient. Absolute return to normal may not be accomplished. The patient should understand this. He should be brought actively into the treatment program, especially in the matter of modifying his chewing habits to bring them more in line with the functional capability of his masticatory apparatus. This requires the selection of softer foods, taking smaller bites, and using slower chewing movements.

Guidelines for Definitive Therapy

In addition to palliative therapy and measures to eliminate cause, appropriate treatment guidelines for the various disorders identified and classified in chapter 8 (see Table 8–1) will be listed. It should be recognized that the individual case may not respond to all the principles proposed. It requires the special attention of the therapist to adapt the principles outlined to meet the circumstances of a particular problem.

If a particular complaint represents more than a single temporomandibular disorder (and many of them do), it is necessary to modify and combine suggestions in the various guidelines to meet the requirements of the case. Also to be considered are transitional phases in masticatory conditions, which require clinical judgment for the selection of the most appropriate course of therapeutic action.

Serious workers in this field should be well informed on all philosophies of management, all concepts of function and dysfunction, and all modalities of treatment, for something is to be learned from each, with perhaps something to be utilized. It should be obvious that the more rational the therapy, the more effective it likely will be. Rational therapy reflects an understanding of basics: functional anatomy, critical standards for judging abnormality, dependable criteria for evaluating symptoms, and techniques for establishing a confirmed diagnosis. Fortunately, the dental literature now has a wealth of source material which can be drawn upon to supply this important information.[1–19]

OCCLUSAL DISHARMONY AND OCCLUSAL CORRECTION.—Many temporomandibular disorders are related etiologically to occlusal disharmony. Many are not. Occlusal disharmony may be a predisposing factor that requires activation by other factors before it becomes a decisive cause. The mere identification of disharmony in the dentition is no assurance that such abnormality is etiologic. It may be irrelevant. It may be symptomatic. Before definitive treatment of the dentition is undertaken, care should be exercised to determine whether the discrepancy is acute (symptomatic) or chronic (preexistent and possibly etiologic), or both. *The safe guideline is to postpone all definitive measures, such as equilibration, alteration, restoration, or reconstruction, until normalization of the muscles and, if possible, the joints.* In the meantime, if correction of the occlusion is needed, it is better to use temporary reversible measures, such as occlusal splinting. When the component of acute malocclusion has been eliminated, it is possible to determine with greater accuracy what needs to be done on a definitive level.

If the dentition is at fault, it must have its effect during power strokes and/or maximum intercuspation, which may be either functional for masticatory purposes or parafunctional due to bruxism. Muscle action is influenced by the dentition from the time the peridontal receptors are stimulated at the beginning of a power stroke until intercuspation is achieved and released. The joint proper is influenced by changes in interarticular pressure induced by power strokes and maximum intercuspation. Finally, the decisive effect of tooth form and position on the joints and musculature is greatest during maximum intercuspation—clenching the teeth in closed position. It is important that discrepancies be identified and taken into account therapeutically. *In these guidelines, however, only temporary occlusal splinting will be suggested when occlusal therapy is indicated. The manner of definitive occlusal therapy will be left to the judgment of the therapist.*

THERAPY FOR ACUTE MUSCLE DISORDERS

Although therapy for each of the three clinically identifiable acute muscle disorders will be listed separately, transitional phases between these disorders are commonplace.

Masticatory Muscle Splinting

In addition to the elimination of cause, the proper treatment for muscle splinting is restriction of use and institution of muscle-relaxant therapy. Chewing should be minimized, for that is what muscle splinting is trying to say: "Stop using me!" Exercises and physiotherapy are contraindicated, as a general rule.

Masticatory Muscle Spasm (MPD Syndromes)

If etiologic factors have been eliminated (or no longer exist), the following principles should resolve a masticatory muscle spasm quickly (7 to 14 days):

1. *Voluntary restriction of all jaw use within painless limits.* Whatever

hurts, don't do! Since it is the pain of use (contracting or stretching the spastic muscle) that has so much to do with perpetuating the spasm, this is an essential first step toward resolving it. This requires understanding and complete cooperation on the part of the patient. Restriction of jaw use must be voluntary; it cannot be imposed by such measures as ligation of the teeth, because that does not prevent contraction of elevator muscles or stretching of lateral pterygoids.

2. *The muscles should be used to the maximum painless limit.* This may seem paradoxical and conflictory, but it is not. Normal use and painless stretching stimulate muscle spindles and Golgi tendon organs, thus reducing activity in the muscle. The continuance of normal painless use is essential to normalization of the muscle. The trick is to properly combine these two principles, both of which are voluntary and require good insight and complete cooperation on the part of the patient. The muscles should not be exercised so much as being put to normal, but painless, use. As pain disappears, the amount of use should be increased gradually until full normal functioning is reestablished. This occurs as spastic activity disappears.

3. *The occlusion should be disengaged.* By disengagement is meant that the tooth surfaces should not be brought into full occlusion. This is to shut off sensory input initiated by the teeth, whether there is occlusal disharmony or not, because it is this input that has much to do with initiating splinting and spastic activity in the first place. It also temporarily arrests all conflicts between the dentition and musculature, whether chronic or acute. Again, it is necessary to have the full cooperation of the patient. This usually can be accomplished voluntarily by simply leaving the teeth apart or ajar. At least, this is true during the waking hours.

If bruxing takes place during the sleeping hours, additional help likely will be needed. Sleeping flat on the back without a pillow may suffice. To this can be added positive autosuggestion: "I will not clench my teeth while I sleep!" Additional support is available in the form of nighttime muscle-relaxant therapy. This is done best by starting at bedtime with a small dose of commonly used relaxant (such as diazepam, $2^{1}/_{2}$ mg) and then estimating its effect the following morning. None is used in the daytime. Then, each night add to the dose until enough effect is obtained that the patient still is able to arouse himself and attend to his duties, *but does so reluctantly.* This should be his maximum dose without interfering with daytime activities also. If such measures fail to eliminate nighttime bruxism, a night-guard appliance of some type should be used. The voluntary method aided with muscle relaxants is better because any type of splinting device encroaches on the interocclusal clearance (freeway space) that may already be minimal due to muscle spasm activity and increased emotional tension. Nor does splinting prevent contraction of elevator muscles. If a nighttime appliance is used, it should be constructed so that it anchors the occlusion at the resting closed position (see Appendix) with the least separation of the teeth. As muscle normalization occurs and acute malocclusion disappears, the device will need to be adjusted by grinding off the occlusal matrix and replacing it in the new occlusal relationship. A disengaging splint should be checked for correctness every 2 to 3 days and altered as needed. When the muscles normalize, it will be noted that further occlusal change ceases.

4. *Interrupt the cycling myospastic activity by analgesic blocking.* The offending muscle(s) should be infiltrated with plain aqueous local anesthetic solution according to the technique suggested in chapter 9, unless there is some specific contraindication. During the period of anesthesia, pain input is shut off, and the muscle can be *massaged gently and manipulated* by stretching and contracting against resistance. This has an excellent normalizing effect without causing pain which would otherwise attend such therapy. The duration of benefit from this treatment should be compared with the known time of anesthesia. If the benefit is of considerably longer duration than the time of anesthesia, then it should be repeated at 48- to 72-hour intervals. If no benefit occurs, repetition is not indicated. If such therapy noticeably increases the symptoms (pain and dysfunction), it may be assumed that inflammatory changes are under way. The diagnosis should then be changed to *myositis*, and the treatment altered accordingly.

When analgesic blocking cannot be done due to specific contraindication or refusal on the patient's part, an alternative method may be substituted. This consists of the use of a vapocoolant, such as Fluori-Methane Spray (Gebauer Chemical Company, Cleveland, Ohio), combined with massage and manipulation. While the offending muscle is under moderate stretch, the overlying skin is streaked with the vapocoolant, holding the nozzle about 12 to 14 inches away. This is repeated several times at intervals of a minute or so. Then, while the pain of spasm is obtunded by the intermittent stimulation of the cutaneous receptors, the muscle is massaged gently and manipulated by stretching and contracting against resistance. This kind of therapy may be repeated as the benefit justifies. It should be understood that the value of vapocoolant therapy is not that of topical anesthesia, and the surface skin should not be frosted.

5. *Postpone definitive therapy until spastic activity is eliminated.* Permanent correction of the occlusion and definitive measures directed toward the muscles or joints should be withheld until the pain and dysfunction symptoms caused by muscle spasm activity have been relieved.

A correctly diagnosed and treated masticatory muscle spasm should resolve quickly and completely in a few days because nothing irreversible is wrong with the muscle. As soon as the CNS impulses that cause the contraction are shut off, the muscle relaxes and symptoms disappear.

If Class III interference symptoms are part of the complaint and are initiated by increased passive interarticular pressure due to continued contraction of elevator muscles, such interference also will disappear as the spastic activity is relieved. If there is persistent interference after the spasm is resolved, then such interference (a) is preexistent, (b) represents the activation of an otherwise dormant, nonsymptomatic interference disorder of the joint, or (c) represents damage to the joint as a result of the muscle spasm. *Interference that persists after resolution of the muscle spasm requires revision of the diagnosis and therapy planned accordingly.*

If the spasm resolves with proper therapy and then promptly recurs when therapy ceases, it should be evident that the etiologic factors responsible for it are still active. This indicates that the diagnosis is incomplete or inaccurate in that it does not properly identify the cause. Two likely possibilities should be investigated: (a) continued input of sensory and/or proprioceptive impulses from the dentition, muscles, or joints due to functional disharmony, and (b) continued input of deep-pain impulses somewhere in the head and neck that is inducing secondary central excitatory effects. Until such cause is located and eliminated, continued therapy for the myospasm will produce only temporary results.

If the spasm fails to respond quickly, there is something wrong with the diagnosis or treatment, or both. It may be that myositis, rather than myospasm, is present. It may be that the condition is really an inflammatory disorder of the joint, and the muscle symptoms are only central excitatory effects. If may be that the treatment has not shut off the central impulses that provoke the spasm. It may be that injudicious treatment is perpetuating the spasm.

The crux of the matter is that if an MPD syndrome cannot be resolved completely and without relapse within a few days, something is wrong with the diagnosis or the treatment, and further efforts are needed to determine what is wrong. All continued therapy should be palliative until the cause for failure has been identified and corrected.

Masticatory Muscle Inflammation (Myositis)

When a masticatory muscle becomes inflamed, a different regimen of therapy is needed. What quickly normalizes a myospasm may aggravate myositis. The principles of therapy for masticatory myositis, in addition to the elimination of cause, include the following:

1. Restriction of jaw use until pain and acute inflammatory symptoms subside. Exercises, stretching the muscle, and injections of the muscle with a local anesthetic are *contraindicated*.

2. Antibiotic therapy and other medical and surgical supportive care are indicated if infection is the chief cause of the inflammation.

3. The judicious use of deep-heat therapy, such as diathermy or ultrasound, is usually beneficial.

4. Nonsteroid anti-inflammatory medications may help resolve the inflammation. These should be employed with medical consent or supervision, especially when used for an extended period of time.

5. As pain and the acute inflammatory symptoms subside, exercises should be instituted, care being taken to *keep them below a painful level*. If such therapy seems to aggravate the condition, it should be minimized or postponed for a while. Such exercises should gradually be increased in frequency and vigor as resolution takes place. Eventually, this should become the dominant feature of therapy.

6. Toward the end of resolution, two considerations warrant attention: *(a)* frequent *momentary* stretching of the muscle should be done to reverse myostatic contracture that may have occurred during the extended time when the muscle was immobilized by inflammation, and *(b)* added exercises consisting of muscle contraction against resistance should be done to rebuild the strength of the muscle lost through atrophic change that results from disuse.

All exercise therapy should be employed with judgment, taking care that it is not excessive or injurious to the healing muscle. *Muscle fatigue must be avoided*. Injudicious physiotherapy may perpetuate and worsen the condition. Perhaps the most important feature of treating myositis is good understanding on the part of the patient concerning its cause, expected behavior, and treatment problems that exist. No shortcuts are available. *Overzealous therapy may be harmful*. Resolution follows an inflammatory curve. Patience is required because the process may be slow—weeks and months, compared with days for myospasm. The muscular dysfunction usually outlasts the pain.

The most serious residual problem after resolution of the inflammation is muscular contracture. If it is myostatic, it usually can be reversed. Myofibrotic contracture, however, may be lasting.

THERAPY FOR DISC-INTERFERENCE DISORDERS

Careful diagnosis is required to classify properly the interference that occurs during jaw movements—the chief symptom of such disorders of the joint. Etiology should be identified and eliminated if possible.

Interference disorders may occur as painless, dormant, nonsymptomatic conditions of which the patient may be quite unaware. Many times such conditions are noticed by the dentist first. They may represent various types of discrete complaints, with and without an element of pain. They suddenly may become activated or seriously aggravated by trauma, emotional stress, or spastic activity in elevator masticatory muscles. They may complicate other joint complaints, such as acute muscle disorders and inflammatory joint conditions. They may develop into inflammatory degenerative arthritis.

After acute muscle conditions, interference disorders of the joint are the most frequent temporomandibular complaint. Interference during jaw movements includes (1) *abnormal sensations,* such as a feeling of rubbing, binding, or catching, (2) *abnormal sounds,* such as clicking, popping, snapping, or grating noise, (3) *abnormal movements,* such as rough, irregular, slipping, catching, or jumping movements, or deviations of the incisal path, and (4) *pain* (if any) that relates in timing to the other symptoms of interference. The ultimate in interference is locking of the joint due to disc jamming or blockage by an anteriorly dislocated articular disc.

Class I Interference

Class I interference disorders cause symptoms in the closed-joint relationship. They occur with clenching the teeth firmly from the unclenched closed-joint position. The primary etiologic factor is occlusal disharmony that induces or permits movement of the disc-condyle complex during maximum intercuspation. Bruxism and habitual excessively hard biting are activating factors. The symptoms can be prevented temporarily by biting against a separator between the teeth.

Treatment for this disorder is correction of the occlusion. This should be done temporarily by using an extremely thin occlusal splint (see Appendix). When it has been properly confirmed that such correction does eliminate the symptoms, definitive correction of the occlusion is needed.

Class II Interference

The symptoms of Class II disc interference occur following maximum intercuspation of the teeth, just as the translatory cycle begins. It also may occur with the first movement after a period of jaw inactivity. Some modified repeat of symptoms may occur if a power stroke ends in maximum intercuspation. The symptoms are timed to the first few millimeters of opening (8 to 10 mm). The primary etiologic factor is occlusal disharmony. Trauma sustained while the teeth are occluded, bruxism, and habitual excessive biting force are other etiologic factors. The symptoms are averted by an occlusal stop that prevents return of the disc-condyle complex to the closed position.

In addition to the elimination of etiologic factors, treatment consists of preventing the disc-condyle complex from returning to closed position for a period of time long enough for natural resolution to repair the damaged surfaces that cause sticking of the articular disc after maximum intercuspation. This is done best by constructing an occlusal splint (see Appendix). Usually, it is necessary only to increase the vertical dimension a few millimeters. Occasionally, however, slight protrusion is required to keep vertical dimension within tolerable limits. A properly constructed splint will prevent the symptoms, yet establish a secure, comfortable, stable occlusal matrix that is satisfactory for chewing purposes. *It must be used 24 hours a day for an extended period of time.* When the patient has been symptom-free for 3 to 4 months, it is well to start adjusting the splint at about 30-day intervals for the purpose of reducing its artificial influence on the patient's occlusion, but without relapse of the complaint. To do this, grind down the occlusal matrix portion of the splint until the symptoms return. Then, add a thin layer of rapid-curing acrylic *sufficient to arrest the symptoms* and create a new occlusal matrix. This step-by-step procedure should continue monthly as long as progress is made in reducing the thickness of the occlusal stop or until the splint is eliminated entirely, which is the ideal objective of therapy. If after several months a plateau of improvement is reached and no further reduction in thickness of the splint can be made without return of the symptoms, permanent alteration of the occlusion in the splinted relationship is indicated. This can be done by permanent splinting (metallic), occlusal onlays, occlusal reconstruction, or orthodontic treatment. One method that warrants consideration is to make a metallic splint and use it long enough to test for correctness. Then, cut off a posterior segment on one side to permit drifting together of two molar teeth. When these come into occlusion and are equilibrated for good contact, cut off a similar segment on the other side and follow the same procedure. This step-by-step removal of the splint should continue until a new occlusal relationship is established in the splinted closed position, and the splint is eliminated completely. Whatever method is used for permanent alteration of the occluded relationship of the teeth should duplicate the splinted position exactly.

Class III Interference

The symptoms of Class III disc interference occur during the course of normal translatory cycles. (This interference does not include symptoms that occur as a result of excessive opening of the mouth or strained movements.) Three basic etiologic situations account for disorders of this type, namely, excessive passive interarticular pressure, structural incompatibility of the sliding surfaces of the joint, and impairment of disc-condyle complex function. Guidelines for the treatment of each of these groups will be considered.

EXCESSIVE PASSIVE INTERARTICULAR PRESSURE.—The best clinical indication that the condition relates to this cause is the temporal behavior of the symptoms: sudden onset, variation, recurrence, relapse. If the symptoms occur in conjunction with an MPD syndrome, it is likely that spasm of elevator muscles is the cause, and treatment for the spasm should automatically be effective for the discal interference as well. If the condition is due to increased emotional tension, measures to reduce such tension should be effective.

During periods of interference, the patient should voluntarily reduce the speed and force of his chewing movements and modify his diet to minimize the interference and prevent more serious damage to the joint. Muscle-relaxant therapy and biofeedback training are indicated if episodes persist.

STRUCTURAL INCOMPATIBILITY OF THE SLIDING SURFACES.—The best indication that the condition relates to this cause is its pattern of sameness. Other indications are deviation of the midline incisal path with opening and closing, increased interference with faster movements, and a tendency to do hard chewing on the symptomatic side. Treatment for this type of discal interference consists of:

1. Modification of jaw use by habit training. This should include (a) the elimination of abusive habits, mannerisms, and nonessential jaw use, (b) more deliberate, slower, and less forceful chewing strokes, and (c) chewing mainly on the symptomatic side.

2. Habit training to find and develop a purposely deviated path of opening-closing that averts the interference. This is a very useful form of therapy, if properly done. One way is to have the patient slowly open until he begins to *feel* the interference, then stop and move laterally one way and then the other until he can feel his way around the interference. If some such deviated path can be found, then have the patient watch himself make these movements in a mirror until he understands what he is doing. Instruct the patient to practice these deviated opening-closing paths for 15 to 20 minutes several times each day, using the mirror as needed. As time goes on and habit patterns slowly are built up to guide the muscles, the movements should become faster, until he develops enough speed to make chewing efforts with these newly acquired compensatory jaw movements practical. With the interference thus eliminated or minimized, natural resolution at the site of obstruction may reduce further the structural incompatibility that causes it.

3. If the condition becomes intolerable and definitive therapy is required, surgical intervention may be necessary. The most promising operation is an eminectomy. It not only eliminates the structural interference but also reduces the required amount of rotatory movement in the disc-

condyle complex during translatory cycles by decreasing the inclination of the articular eminence.

IMPAIRMENT OF DISC-CONDYLE COMPLEX FUNCTION.—The best clinical indications that the condition relates to this cause are (1) more or less continuous symptoms of interference, such as sensations of rough, irregular movements and grating noise, (2) punctuation of symptoms by discrete noises and disc locking, (3) skidding subluxating movements throughout the translatory cycle, (4) reciprocal functional displacements or dislocations of the disc, (5) associated sensations of ipsilateral overstressed or disoccluded posterior teeth when clenched, (6) protracted dislocation of the disc, and (7) aggravation of symptoms by chewing on the symptomatic side.

Conservative therapeutic efforts for Class III disorders due to impaired disc-condyle complex functioning may not be rewarding. Many times the best that can be done, short of surgical intervention, is to minimize abusive use in order to retard or arrest progressive deterioration and help the patient accept and tolerate an undesirable situation. The following guidelines may be helpful: (1) the patient should be given full insight into the problem and its cause so that he can understand the symptoms better and do his part to help retard progress toward degenerative arthritis, and (2) habit training to make chewing less stressful should be encouraged. This means softer foods, smaller bites, slower and less vigorous chewing movements. It is necessary to eliminate as much as possible all abusive joint use, minimize functional demands, and learn to sense and avoid discrete instances of interference and disc jamming. Palliative treatment to control pain and careful elimination of etiologic factors, *especially chronic occlusal disharmony*, are definitely indicated.

Rational definitive therapy depends chiefly on the accuracy of diagnosis, as follows:

Adhesions Between the Articular Disc and Condyle.—Fibrous adhesions between the articular disc and mandibular condyle eliminate hinge action and induce skid-like subluxated movements throughout the translatory cycles. If the complaint becomes intolerable, surgical intervention is required to remove the articular disc. This may be done by a high condylectomy. Prosthetic replacement is required.

Damaged Articular Disc.—Progressive deterioration of the articular disc may cause continuous rough and noisy translatory movements punctuated by discrete noise and disc jamming at points of greater interference. Fracture of the disc causes a sensation of ipsilateral overstressed posterior teeth during maximum intercuspation if the fragments are separated, or disocclusion if they override each other. If the complaint becomes intolerable, surgical intervention is required to excise the disc and replace it with a prosthetic substitute.

Dysfunctional Discal Ligaments.—Deteriorated, elongated, or detached discal ligaments permit sliding movement in the disc-condyle complex. *Functional displacements of the articular disc* depend on the extent of elongation of the ligaments in conjunction with deterioration of the disc itself. The symptoms relate to abnormal sliding movement between the disc and condyle and consist of noise, irregular movement, and disc jamming. The disc is displaced anteriorly by action of the superior lateral pterygoid muscle as a result of active contraction during power strokes, rapid closure, and maximum intercuspation. It is displaced posteriorly by action of the superior retrodiscal lamina during full forward translatory movement as with opening widely. The timing of the disc noise, therefore, relates to (1) sticking of the disc in the fossa after maximum intercuspation (which causes disc noise during the early phase of opening), (2) opening the mouth widely (which causes disc noise in the later opening effort), (3) power strokes or rapid closure (which cause noise during closing movements), and (4) maximum intercuspation (which causes noise at the end of closing movements or on clenching the teeth). Disc jamming may occur at points of greater interference and, like the other symptoms, relates to such things as passive interarticular pressure, inclination of the articular eminence, speed and force of jaw movement, and the kind of food being chewed. The symptom pattern, therefore, may be quite variable indeed.

Momentary disc jamming is of little consequence. Protracted disc jamming is more serious and should be differentiated from protracted functional dislocation of the disc. Protracted jamming remains relatively silent and painless, causes no acute malocclusion, and may permit disproportionate protrusive and lateral excursive movement. Protracted functional dislocation, in contrast, causes noisy movements, retrodiscitis pain, acute malocclusion during maximum intercuspation, and proportionate restriction of protrusive and lateral movements.

To relieve protracted disc jamming, the mandible should be manipulated gently from side to side. Biting against resistance on the symptomatic side may relieve it. Forceful opening, however, should be avoided.

Symptoms that follow maximum intercuspation or clenching the teeth may sometimes be prevented by inserting an occlusal stop between the teeth. Conservative treatment consisting of an occlusal splint that prevents the condyle from returning to its fully occluded position may be beneficial. Although a splint that increases vertical dimension may prove effective, if it tends to exceed resting position, it may not be tolerated by the patient. Therefore, the best results are usually obtained by a splint that holds the mandible in a slightly protruded position. If such a splint is effective, this type of therapy should be pursued as far as seems practical. But, if permanent occlusal correction based on temporary splinting is contemplated, it is wise to try a test period without the splint, to see if relapse promptly occurs (which it should, if the device really arrests the symptoms). It should be noted, however, that splinting sometimes aggravates the symptoms.

Functional dislocation of the articular disc may occur when deterioration of the anterior or posterior portion of the disc is sufficient to permit its being drawn through the articular disc space and the discal ligaments are sufficiently elongated to permit such gross displacement. Anterior dislocation occurs during a power stroke, *especially on the biting side*, and reciprocal reduction automatically occurs with a full forward translatory movement (opening widely). Posterior dislocation occurs with opening the mouth widely, and reciprocal functional reduction automatically takes place during a power stroke or full closure. The patient, therefore, should be taught to recognize such dislocations and how to maneuver reduction. If the dislocation takes place during a power stroke or maximum intercuspation, he should reduce it by opening widely. If the dislocation occurs during opening or protrusion, he should reduce it by biting hard on an object placed between the teeth *on the affected side*. It should be noted that anterior dislocations require full forward translation to effect functional reduction. If such movement becomes blocked by the dislocated disc, reduction is prevented. He should then try to maneuver the jaw open by deviating from side to side. If by so doing, he is able to open widely, reduction occurs. Otherwise, it remains as protracted dislocation. During such a time, the patient should avoid bringing the teeth into full maximum intercuspation. Protracted posterior functional dislocation does not occur.

Prevention of functional dislocation is important to the patient. The incidence of anterior dislocation is reduced by chewing on the opposite side, avoiding hard objects and large bites, and avoiding bringing the teeth into firm maximum intercuspation. The incidence of posterior dislocation is reduced by avoiding full opening and extended protrusive movements.

For the treatment of functional displacement and/or dislocation of the articular disc, the judicious use of sclerosing therapy is justified. Because of possible anaphylactoid reaction, caution should be used. With the joint properly anesthetized with a local anesthetic, an injection of 1 ml of 5% sodium morrhuate is deposited in the lateral wall of the capsular ligament. The joint should then be immobilized by intermaxillary fixation for about 14 days following the injection. If the results seem to justify it, the treatment may be repeated in 30 days. The objective is to tighten the capsular ligament by the proliferation of fibrous tissue and, thus, reduce movement between the disc and condyle during translatory cycles. If sclerosing does not control the symptoms and the complaint requires definitive treatment, surgical intervention is required. Arthroplasty is usually the operation of choice in which the articular disc and condyle are sutured more tightly together. Sometimes the results are improved by doing an eminectomy also. In case of protracted functional dislocation, distortion and deformation of the disc may require surgical intervention. If the articular disc is excised, prosthetic replacement is needed to forestall later occlusal problems due to collapse of the articular disc space.

Dysfunctional Superior Retrodiscal Lamina.—A nonfunctional superior retrodiscal lamina eliminates the only intracapsular source of posterior traction on the articular disc. In such case, anterior dislocation of the articular disc, whether it be traumatic, spontaneous, or functional, is *permanent*. Surgical intervention is the only form of effective therapy.

Class IV Interference

The symptoms of Class IV interference occur during overextension of opening beyond the limits of normal rotation in the disc-condyle complex. This condition is referred to usually as subluxation (partial or incomplete dislocation) or joint hypermobility. The cause is habitual overextension of mouth opening.

The treatment for Class IV disorders is habit training to restrict mouth opening within normal limits. This usually can be accomplished by voluntary restraint on the part of the patient. Sometimes a training device is very helpful. This consists of placing Ivy eyelets or ligating jeweler loops at each of the four first bicuspid teeth. Then tie a piece of 6-pound monofilament nylon fishing cord to the right mandibular loop and pass it up through the right maxillary loop, across and down through the left maxillary loop, and through the left mandibular loop. Then open the mouth to a point just short of the subluxating symptoms and tie off the nylon cord at the left mandibular loop (Fig 10–1). This device does not interfere with normal opening and chewing. When excessive opening is attempted, however, the cord arrests it. The device should be used for several weeks, until the restricted opening becomes habitual. The patient should be taught how to replace the nylon cord to the measured opening proper for his case, because it is chewed through in a few days.

If such habit training fails and the condition becomes intolerable, sclerosing therapy may be tried. True definitive treatment, however, is surgical. This is best done by eminectomy. The operation flattens the articular eminence and reduces the amount of posterior rotation required for a full forward translatory movement. By so doing, the rotatory movement in the

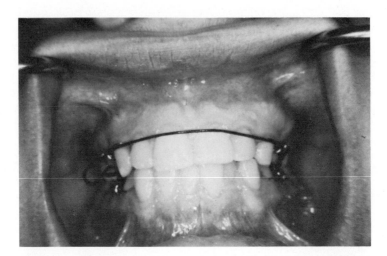

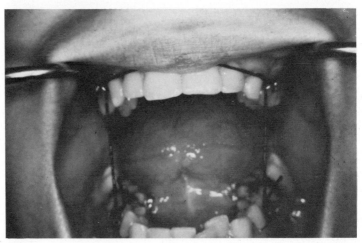

Fig 10–1.—Simple restraining device limits the extent of mouth opening for the purpose of training the musculature to control habitual excessive opening of the mouth. *Top,* an Ivy eyelet or jeweler loop is placed at the mesial of the maxillary first bicuspid teeth and between the mandibular bicuspid teeth. A nylon cord (6-pound monofilament nylon fishing cord) is tied to the right mandibular loop, passed up through the right maxillary, across and down through the left maxillary, and on through the left mandibular loop. The mouth is opened to the desired point of restraint and the cord drawn tight and tied off at the left mandibular loop. *Bottom,* mouth opened to the maximum permitted by the restraining device. Within the imposed limit there is satisfactory freedom of mandibular movement.

disc-condyle complex no longer exceeds normal limits, and arrested movement of the disc on the condyle does not take place. After the operation, extended opening does not cause subluxation.

Spontaneous Anterior Dislocation

If at the moment of full or extended opening, the articular disc is forced through the articular disc space by an overextended opening, or if there is premature contraction of the superior lateral pterygoid muscle, the disc loses contact with the articular eminence; the disc space collapses; the condyle moves up against the articular eminence; and the disc is trapped in front of the condyle. With the articular disc space collapsed, the superior retrodiscal lamina cannot rotate the trapped disc posteriorly. When effort is made to close, the superior lateral pterygoid muscle contracts simultaneously with the elevator muscles, thus prolapsing the disc forward on the condyle. The dislocated disc remains anterior to the condyle and normal closure is blocked. The posterior teeth strike, while the anteriors stand widely apart.

To reduce a spontaneously dislocated articular disc, all that is needed is to widen the collapsed articular disc space just enough to permit the stretched superior retrodiscal lamina to rotate the disc back into position on the condyle. When such space is provided, reduction is automatic. Contraction of the superior lateral pterygoid muscle prevents reduction. Since this muscle contracts simultaneously with elevator muscles, any maneuver that entails contraction of elevator muscles (biting force) also prevents reduction; the contracted superior lateral pterygoid muscle nullifies the elastic traction of the stretched superior retrodiscal lamina that is essential to such reduction. Any such maneuver, therefore, is contraindicated.

Acute spontaneous anterior dislocation.—To reduce acute dislocation, relaxation of elevator and superior lateral pterygoid muscles is needed to widen the collapsed articular disc space. This is done best by having the patient yawn as widely as he can. At that moment, slight posterior pressure on the chin is usually enough to accomplish reduction. If a little more space is needed, pressing the mandible downward with the thumbs on the external oblique ridges *while the patient yawns* will suffice. A patient can be taught this maneuver to reduce his own dislocations. Forced attempts at reduction by the patient or the doctor may complicate the situation considerably. Forced reduction tends to initiate myospasm activity in the elevator muscles, making widening of the collapsed articular disc space all the more difficult. If this should take place, local anesthesia of the spastic muscles usually will facilitate reduction. Myospasm of the lateral pterygoid muscle renders reduction impossible. If this should occur, local anesthesia of that muscle is mandatory, or a general anesthetic with succinylcholine chloride muscle relaxant may become necessary.

RECURRENT SPONTANEOUS ANTERIOR DISLOCATION.—When spontaneous anterior dislocation occurs frequently, the patient should be taught how to reduce it effectively without introducing complications caused by the use of force. It is better, however, that it be prevented. This condition is the result of habitually opening the mouth too wide and almost always is a complication of chronic subluxation. Most such patients can be trained to open less widely and, therefore, eliminate both the Class IV interference and the occasional spontaneous dislocation. This can be done by utilizing the habit-training device described for the management of chronic subluxation. If the condition is not controlled by habit training and becomes intolerable, thus requiring definitive therapy, surgical intervention is needed. The operation best suited to eliminate this condition is an eminectomy, because it flattens the articular eminence and thus reduces the amount of posterior rotation of the articular disc during forward translatory movements. When the amount of discal rotation is reduced, normal forward limits of the translatory cycle are extended, and subluxation and spontaneous anterior dislocation do not take place with full opening movements.

CHRONIC ANTERIOR DISLOCATION.—Chronic anterior dislocation of the temporomandibular joint is due to (1) contracture of the lateral pterygoid muscle, (2) permanent prolapse of the articular disc from a nonfunctional superior retrodiscal lamina, or (3) healed fracture-dislocation following trauma. Correction of this condition calls for surgical intervention. Several operations are used depending on the particular problem at hand, namely, myotomy of the lateral pterygoid muscle, eminectomy, arthroplasty, and reconstructive surgery.

THERAPY FOR INFLAMMATORY DISORDERS

Therapeutic guidelines for capsulitis, retrodiscitis, and inflammatory arthritis will be listed. When the complaint represents a combination of these disorders, considerable clinical judgment is needed for proper treatment planning.

Capsulitis and Synovitis

Capsulitis occurring as a separate entity usually is due to trauma. The majority of cases displaying symptoms of capsulitis are secondary to other inflammatory conditions arising as the result of injury to the discal collateral ligaments or the temporomandibular ligament. Some are secondary to inflammatory arthritis, periarticular conditions, or injury to a preexistent capsular fibrosis. Etiology usually entails the identification of other types of disorders. Consequently, therapy may be directed toward conditions besides the capsulitis per se.

In general, the treatment for capsulitis and synovitis includes:

1. Restriction of condylar movements that tend to stretch the capsule.

2. Deep-heat therapy using diathermy or ultrasound.

3. Anti-inflammatory medications. If the capsulitis is due to trauma and not likely to be repeated, a single injection of corticosteroid made laterally to the capsular ligament is usually effective.

4. Special considerations are needed if the capsulitis is secondary to other disorders: (a) If the capsulitis accompanies pain that is reduced by biting against a separator, it likely relates to inflamed discal ligaments or temporomandibular ligament. Occlusal correction with a temporary occlusal splint is indicated (see Appendix). Permanent correction may be planned when the capsulitis has subsided. (b) If the capsulitis is due to periarticular inflammation, active treatment of the primary condition, including antibiotics and supportive medical and surgical care, may be needed. (c) If the capsulitis is a manifestation of inflammatory arthritis, treatment should be directed primarily toward the arthritic condition.

Retrodiscitis

Many inflammatory conditions of the retrodiscal tissue result from extrinsic trauma of a type that could have caused a mandibular fracture. The diagnosis usually is made only after a futile radiographic search for a fracture line. Since hemarthrosis may be present, treatment should take into account the prevention, if possible, of ankylosis. The treatment for this kind of retrodiscitis entails:

1. Intermaxillary fixation to establish normal occlusal relations.

2. Periodic release of the fixation and active movement of the joint for 5 to 10 minutes at least twice daily.

3. As soon as the occlusion will remain stabilized without the aid of intermaxillary fixation, active movement of the joint should be encouraged until resolution is complete.

If the retrodiscitis occurs insidiously as a result of injury to the retrodiscal tissue (due to nonanchored posterior overclosure), occlusal correction is needed. If due to protracted functional dislocation, surgical intervention may be required.

Inflammatory Arthritis

The symptoms of generalized inflammation of the joint are much the same, regardless of cause. Therefore, certain general principles of treatment may apply to all types. As the particular kind of arthritis becomes evident, special considerations are needed. The following therapeutic principles are usually indicated:

1. Functional demands should be reduced voluntarily to bring them well within the capabilities of the inflamed joint.

2. Nonpainful movements of the joint should be maintained on a periodic schedule of 5 to 10 minutes two to three times daily to keep the joint mobile. This should not be carried to the point of pain or other sign of aggravation of the inflammatory condition.

3. Acute malocclusion and other obvious discrepancies in occlusal function should be corrected by occlusal disengagement (see Masticatory Muscle Spasm therapy). If an occlusal splint is used, it should be corrected periodically as resolution or further deterioration takes place.

4. Medically supervised anti-inflammatory medications and other supportive medical treatment usually are indicated.

5. Judicious physiotherapy in the form of deep heat (diathermy or ultrasound) should be used unless it seems to aggravate the condition.

6. Since inflammatory arthritis frequently causes arthralgic pain of a more or less continuous type, some secondary central excitatory effects may accompany the disorder and complicate the symptom picture. Secondary referred pains and muscle spasm activity should be identified. The referred pain will remain dependent on the arthralgia, but muscle spasm activity may become an independent cycling pain-dysfunction syndrome that requires separate management (see Therapy for Acute Muscle Disorders). It should be understood that, until the arthralgia is eliminated or at least brought to the stage of intermittency, lasting resolution of such muscle spasm activity cannot be expected.

7. Some special considerations depend on the kind of arthritis present. *Degenerative arthritis* may require special management of the dentition using principles suggested under Disc-Interference Disorders of the Joint. Surgical intervention may be required, such as closed condylotomy or arthroplasty. Good postsurgical care and follow-up are essential to satisfactory management of the case. *Rheumatoid arthritis* is essentially a medical problem. The dentist's responsibility rests largely with adjusting the occlusion as necessary. Progressive loss of contact of the anterior teeth may require occlusal splinting, adjusted periodically as further change takes place. Reconstructive arthroplasty may be needed. *Traumatic and infectious arthritis* may require antibiotic therapy as well as general supportive medical and surgical care. Caution should be exercised to minimize undesirable sequelae, if possible. *Hyperuricemia* is a medical problem requiring active treatment and follow-up. Since it follows a recurring pattern, continuing medical supervision is needed.

8. Corticosteroid therapy may have a place in the treatment program,

but considerable judgment should be exercised in its use. It is frequently part of rheumatoid arthritis treatment. Injections of corticosteroid substances into the joint proper may be justified at times. It is known to predispose to further deterioration and encourages excessive use of the joint during the time that it suppresses the inflammation. When it has been established that a surgical approach to degenerative arthritis is to be made, periodic injections of corticosteroid into the joint may be used to keep the patient comfortable pending surgery.

THERAPY FOR CHRONIC MANDIBULAR HYPOMOBILITIES

Usually, no treatment of any kind is needed for chronic mandibular hypomobilities, unless they are injured by movements that exceed the limitations imposed and, thus, cause inflammation to develop. Good management of all chronic hypomobilities includes adequate insight into the problem on the patient's part, so he may be able to avoid abusive use of the joint. Careful habit training to keep all joint functioning well within the structural capabilities of the joint is needed. Care should be exercised by the dentist to avoid opening the mouth too widely. It should be understood that the opposite joint should be kept under observation, because the restricted movements in the hypomobile joint may cause destructive changes in the mobile joint.

Contractured Elevator Muscle

Extracapsular chronic mandibular hypomobility due to muscular contracture may become inflamed due to excessive opening efforts. As such, it should be treated as *myositis,* until the acute symptoms subside.

Myostatic contracture.—If contracture is due to protracted restriction of opening, it may usually be reversed with proper therapy. This consists of *gentle momentary stretching* of the muscle several times each day. Stretching should not be great enough to cause pain or forceful enough to cause muscle inflammation. It should be just enough to stimulate the inverse stretch reflex. Many weeks are required for the resting length of the muscle to be increased.

It should be noted that myostatic contracture may complicate other kinds of chronic mandibular hypomobility, especially myofibrotic contracture and ankylosis. This is to be considered when other forms are under treatment. Even though correction of such other disorders is properly planned and executed, provision should be made in the postsurgical treatment regimen for the reversal of any accompanying myostatic contracture that may be present.

MYOFIBROTIC CONTRACTURE.—If the contracture is due to the formation of cicatricial tissue in and about the muscle, the shortening is permanent. Mild but continuous elastic traction to lengthen the muscle by linear growth may accomplish some degree of benefit. If definitive treatment is required, surgical detachment and reattachment is necessary.

It should be noted that myofibrotic contracture of long standing may be complicated by myostatic contracture of the other elevator muscles. If this is so, treatment should include staging in such a way that the myofibrotic contractured muscle is detached. Then treatment for the myostatic contractured muscles should be accomplished before the reattachment procedure is completed.

Capsular Fibrosis

Capsular fibrosis restricts movement in the outer ranges only and usually poses no intolerable condition that requires definitive treatment. The usual problem is merely that of injury induced by excessive force used to extend condylar movement. As such, the injured capsule becomes inflamed, and the condition should be treated as a *capsulitis*.

Ankylosis

The usual form of ankylosis is fibrous, in which adhesions join the disc-condyle complex to the articular eminence-fossa surface. Forceful movements may injure the adhesions, thus causing pain and inflammation. Treatment consists of voluntary restraint of joint use until the inflammatory condition subsides. Anti-inflammatory medications and deep-heat therapy (diathermy or ultrasound) are usually beneficial. Exercises are contraindicated.

Ordinarily a 25-mm opening can be made, whether the condition is fibrous or osseous. If a larger opening is required and the complaint becomes intolerable, surgery is necessary. Good postsurgical care and follow-up are essential to satisfactory final results.

Ankylosis may be complicated by myostatic contracture of several or all elevator muscles due to the protracted inability to open the mouth normally. This complicates the diagnosis as well as the treatment. When it is determined that such contracture exists, provision for the normalization of the contractured muscles should be included in the treatment plan.

THERAPY FOR DISORDERS OF GROWTH

Disorders of growth involving the craniomandibular articulation usually occur insidiously. Compensatory changes occur in such a manner that little or no pain or dysfunction becomes evident until the condition is well developed. Such disorders are usually apparent radiographically before symptoms develop enough to require definitive therapy.

Aberrations related to the developmental process, acquired changes in structural form, and benign neoplasia usually require interdisciplinary planning and corrective treatment that embraces surgery, orthodontics, rehabilitation efforts, and cosmetic procedures. Malignancy involving the joint requires the services of a consulting oncologist.

REFERENCES

1. Alling C.C. III, Mahan P.E. (eds.): *Facial Pain,* ed. 2. Philadelphia, Lea & Febiger, 1977.
2. Bell W.E.: *Temporomandibular Joint Disease.* Dallas, Egan Company Press, 1960.
3. Bell W.E.: *Synopsis: Oral and Facial Pain and The Temporomandibular Joint.* Dallas, Welden E. Bell, Publisher, 1967.
4. Bell W.E.: *Orofacial Pains: Differential Diagnosis,* ed. 2. Chicago, Year Book Medical Publishers, 1979.
5. Dubner R., Sessle B.J., Storey A.T.: *The Neural Basis of Oral and Facial Function,* New York, Plenum Press, 1978.
6. Du Brul E.L.: *Sicher's Oral Anatomy,* ed. 7. St. Louis, C.V. Mosby Co., 1980.
7. Freese A.S., Scheman P.: *Management of Temporomandibular Joint Problems.* St. Louis, C.V. Mosby Co., 1962.
8. Gelb H. (ed.): *Clinical Management of Head, Neck and TMJ Pain and Dysfunction.* Philadelphia, W.B. Saunders Co., 1977.
9. Irby W.B. (ed.): *Current Advances in Oral Surgery.* St. Louis, C.V. Mosby Co., 1980, vol. 3.
10. Morgan D.H., Hall W.P., Vamvas S.J. (eds.): *Diseases of the Temporomandibular Apparatus.* St. Louis, C.V. Mosby Co., 1977.
11. Sarnat B.G. (ed.): *The Temporomandibular Joint.* Springfield, Ill., Charles C Thomas, Publisher, 1951.
12. Sarnat B.G. (ed.): *The Temporomandibular Joint,* ed. 2. Springfield, Ill., Charles C Thomas, Publisher, 1964.
13. Sarnat B.G., Laskin D.M. (eds.): *The Temporomandibular Joint,* ed. 3. Springfield, Ill., Charles C Thomas, Publisher, 1979.
14. Schwartz L. (ed.): *Diseases of the Temporomandibular Joint.* Philadelphia, W.B. Saunders Co., 1959.
15. Schwartz L., Chayes C.M. (eds.): *Facial Pain and Mandibular Dysfunction.* Philadelphia, W.B. Saunders Co., 1968.
16. Shore N.A.: *Occlusal Equilibration and Temporomandibular Joint Dysfunction.* Philadelphia, J.B. Lippincott Co., 1959.
17. Shore N.A.: *Temporomandibular Joint Dysfunction and Occlusal Equilibration,* ed. 2. Philadelphia, J.B. Lippincott Co., 1976.
18. Solberg W.K., Clark G.T. (eds.): *Temporomandibular Joint Problems.* Chicago, Quintessence Publishing Co., 1980.
19. Zarb G.A., Carlsson G.E. (eds.): *Temporomandibular Joint Function and Dysfunction.* Copenhagen, Munksgaard, 1979.

Appendix

The Occlusal Splint

Various satisfactory methods for constructing occlusal splinting devices are available. The following is a modification of the method originally offered by John R. Thompson.[1]

MAKING THE ACRYLIC SPLINT.—Take an impression of the upper arch and pour a cast. Adapt a single thickness of ordinary baseplate wax to cover the teeth and palate. Trim the wax to include just the incisal edges of the anterior teeth and to a point slightly beyond the greatest contour of the posterior teeth, so that the finished splint will be retained by springing on. (Note: If the splint is for short-term use as a disengaging device, the anterior teeth need not be included.) Process in transparent acrylic and fit to the mouth, being sure that it is securely retained and comfortable (without pressure on the palatal tissues). Remove the acrylic base from the mouth, and grind down the thickness in the occlusal matrix area until holes appear. This is done so that the finished splint will separate the teeth as little as possible. (Note: If the splint is for a measured occlusal stop, this step may not be needed.) Mix some self-curing acrylic material and place a thin layer over the occlusal matrix portion of the base. Place in the patient's mouth, and have him close by *gently resting the teeth together* against the splint. Do not use biting force. Do not guide him. *Let his own relaxed muscles establish the occlusal position*. After a few minutes, remove from the mouth and permit to cure completely. Trim excess material, and smooth any roughness, but leave most of the anchoring occlusal matrix intact.

TESTING THE SPLINT FOR CORRECTNESS.—The finished splint should meet the following criteria:
1. It should feel comfortable and secure in the mouth, with adequate retention.
2. When the teeth are "tap-tapped" lightly against the splint, they should strike simultaneously.
3. When the teeth are clenched firmly against the splint, no movement

---

[1]Thompson J.R.: Temporomandibular disorders: Diagnosis and dental treatment, in Sarnat B.G. (ed.): *The Temporomandibular Joint*. Springfield, Ill., Charles C Thomas, Publisher, 1951, pp. 122–144.

should be sensed, and biting pressure should feel uniform bilaterally.

If any deficiency exists, grind away the added acrylic material, and re-peat the step of adding self-curing material as outlined above. Several such trials may be required to achieve the objective of producing an occlusal matrix that will hold the mandible at the closed resting (unclenched) posi-tion.

CONVERSION OF THE ACRYLIC SPLINT INTO METAL.—Take impressions of both arches, and pour casts. Mount the casts in an articulator, using the acrylic splint as a bite. Wax up for casting in metal. Use minimal bulk; include just the incisal edges of the anterior teeth and the occlusal contact area posteriorly. A palatal bar and clasps should be used for strength and retention. Cast, finish, and adapt to the mouth for comfort and retention. Equilibrate if needed. Mill in the finished splint with abrasive paste for a minute or so to eliminate minute discrepancies and to remove the surface glaze from the occlusal matrix area. Test for correctness as described above.

Note: With steeply inclined articular eminences, the full occlusal matrix as produced usually is quite comfortable and acceptable to the patient. Patients with relatively flat dentitions, however, may feel the occlusion as "too tight." In such cases, it should be eased a little by careful grinding to permit a little more freedom in the occluded position. This applies espe-cially to the anterior teeth.

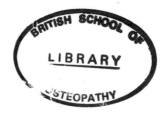

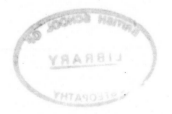

Index